15
BAR

EDINBURGH
EDUCATION AND SOCIETY
SERIES
General Editor: Colin Bell

Authorities
and Partisans

The Debate on Unemployment and Health

MEL BARTLEY

EDINBURGH UNIVERSITY PRESS

© Edinburgh University Press, 1992

Edinburgh University Press
22 George Square, Edinburgh

Set in Linotron Palatino
by Koinonia Ltd, Bury, and
printed in Great Britain by
Hartnoll Ltd, Bodmin

A CIP record for this book is
available from the British Library

ISBN 0 7486 0334 4

CONTENTS

ACKNOWLEDGEMENTS

First of all I must thank Richard Cummins, who made me begin to think it could all be possible. Particular thanks are also due to some of the participants in the debate: Derek Cook, Steve Platt, Jennie Popay, Alex Scott-Samuel, Gill Westcott, Jon Stern, Mike Porter and Steve Engelman, and to all those who kindly agreed to give me their accounts and interpretations of events. There were others whose help also went well beyond the role of interviewees, and my understanding of many issues both scientific and political benefited enormously from my contact with the talented and innovative participants in the unemployment and health debate.

It was my great good luck that Edinburgh University contains both Britain's leading department of social policy and the Science Studies Unit which has pioneered work in the Strong Programme in the sociology of scientific knowledge. I would like to thank Donald Mackenzie for introducing me to much of the literature in the latter area. Moira Forrest was Information Officer in the Unit while I was doing this study and patiently helped me to find my way through this literature. I also greatly appreciated the colleagueship of the Unit's graduate students, especially Ann Elder and Steve Sturdy.

Thanks also to Bryan Christie for allowing me an inside view of how health topics are dealt with in an outstanding newspaper.

Without the intellectual and personal support of friends, and of my fellow graduate students in the Department of Social Policy and Social Work this study would never have seen the light of day. I thank Jim Carnie, Alison Harold, Brian Henderson, Diane Kennedy, Shirley Platz, Erio Ziglio and most especially Liz Jagger, Claudia Martin and David Blane.

The Department of Social Policy provided a stimulating and secure environment throughout the considerable ups and downs involved in this work. It was a privilege to experience Edinburgh's supervisory system, thanks to which I benefited from the expertise of Neil Fraser as my second supervisor. In interdisciplinary studies such as this one, the value of supervision from two people with different disciplinary backgrounds can hardly be stressed enough.

My senior supervisor, Professor Adrian Sinfield, took something of a risk in allowing this study to try and develop such an unlikely link as that between social policy and the sociology of science and technology. For this, and for his guidance and support, my greatest debt is owed to him.

ABBREVIATIONS

BRHS   British Regional Heart Study
CSRC   Chief Scientist's Research Committee
DPH   Diploma in Public Health
DS   Decennial Supplement
EA   Economic Adviser
ESRC   Economic and Social Research Council
GSS   Government Statistical Service
LS   Longitudinal Study
LSHT   London School of Hygiene and Tropical Medicine
MOsH   Medical Officers of Health
MSC   Manpower Services Commission
NCVO   National Council for Voluntary Organisations
OCS   Office of the Chief Scientist
OPCS   Office of Population Censuses and Surveys
POHG   Politics of Health Group
PQ   Parliamentary Question
PSU   Policy Strategy Unit
RPTC   Regional Poisoning Treatment Centre
RSS   Royal Statistical Society
SCM   Specialist in Community Medicine
SHEG   Scottish Health Education Group
SMR   Standardised Mortality Ratio
SCUF   Social Costs of Unemployment Forum
SSK   Sociology of Scientific Knowledge
SSRU   Social Statistics Research Unit
UHSG   Unemployment and Health Study Group
UHSP   Unit for the Study of Health Policy

Part One

The Debate on Unemployment and Health

1

INTRODUCTION: SOCIAL PROBLEMS
AND SCIENTIFIC CONTROVERSY

Controversy around the health effects of high unemployment is
nothing new in Britain. The question of 'physical deterioration'
has a long history in social policy debate (Pfautz 1967, Hennock
1976). It has formed the centre of many political storms over the
adequacy of both wages and levels of benefit. The question of
whether the notion of giving sufficient money to allow 'physical
subsistence' to someone whose labour is not in demand can be
justified within a strict market economy, is an 'essentially contested' one in western industrial societies. This problem is com-
pounded by repeated findings of studies since the early twentieth
century that the lower levels of wages tended to be lower than the
amount needed to pay for a diet prescribed by expert studies as
sufficient to sustain physical health. In the 1970s and 1980s this
problem surfaced in the form of debates over the 'replacement
ratio' (of benefits to wages, see Micklewright 1986, Cooke 1988),
and in the form of 'scrounger scares' (Golding and Middleton
1982; Deacon 1976, 1978; Deacon and Sinfield 1977; Popay 1977),
purporting to show that benefits were too high, and were being
used to support deviant or luxurious lifestyles. It is not therefore
particularly surprising to find a controversy taking place in the
late 1970s and 1980s, as it did in the 1930s (Webster 1982). 'The
health of the unemployed' is the sort of issue which recedes
during times of prosperity and reappears at times of economic
crisis. Such issues may provide good opportunities to study the
relationship between research and policy.

There have been many attempts to discover how research influences policy in post-war Britain and the United States (for
example, Caplan 1976; Rein 1980, 1983; Weiss 1979; Bulmer 1983;
and the various papers collected in Kallen *et al.* 1982, to give but a
few recent examples). Many of these studies have been concerned
with how researchers might increase the influence of their work,
and what kind of research is taken most seriously by policy-

makers. Few, however, have dealt with public health, which is rather surprising in view of the dominance of medical scientists in this sphere – although it may be *because* of this very dominance that the relationship has not been regarded as interesting. The health implications of unemployment has been an exception to this rule. Webster's (1982) paper on 'Healthy or hungry 'Thirties?' has given an account of some of the ways in which different sorts of evidence about the health of the unemployed during the Great Depression were used in policy debate. The present study aims to undertake a similar task for the 1980s.

Some time ago, F. M.Martin remarked that:

> There may be a doctoral thesis to be won by sieving through the products of academic social medicine in order to capture a few specimens of policy-oriented research, and by painfully reconstructing the relevant policy processes. (Martin 1977)

The present study treats the debate on whether unemployment has a deleterious effect on physical (as opposed to mental) health as a case study in the relationship between public health research and economic and social policy. It attempts to reconstruct and make sense of the progress of the debate in order to address some of the questions posed by previous work on the relationship between scientific and policy debates, and to throw light on the apparent paradoxes which arose as the debate unfolded. This is done in two ways: by setting out in some detail the story of how researchers came to be interested in the topic, how they worked on it, and how their results came to the attention of policy-makers; and by analysing this course of events with the help of theoretical perspectives drawn from social policy, the sociology of the media, and the social study of science.

In the course of this exploration, some light is also thrown on the question: 'does unemployment cause ill health or early death? Although this study does not claim to settle that question, it aims to contribute towards our ability to evaluate arguments in this and other similar controversies. During the course of the study it became increasingly clear that anyone who wants to be 'really scientific' needs to be able to stand back from their own and other people's research efforts and understand the context and the processes by which these efforts are shaped.

Both the question 'does unemployment harm health?' and the actions of those who became concerned with it turn out to be rather more complex than most participants in and observers of the debate had anticipated. Therefore, the book is divided into two sections: the first tells the story of the debate; the second carries out a more analytical task. Obviously, however, no 'story' is told without some guiding thread to the narrative, and it would be misleading to imply that the first section of this book is just an account of a sequence of events. 'The effect of unemployment on health' has been treated here as a 'social problem' as defined by sociologists of deviance (for example, Spector and Kitsuse 1977; Downs 1973; Richardson and Jordan 1979 and, for Britain Manning 1985), and the scientific and policy debates around the question are regarded analytically as a 'social problem process'. Because this account focuses more closely on the scientific debate, guiding ideas have also been drawn from two recently developed approaches to studying scientific controversy: the 'Strong Programme' in the sociology of scientific knowledge and the 'translation model' developed in France by Bruno Latour, Michel Callon and their colleagues.

The 'natural' history of social problems

For Spector and Kitsuse, social problems are not in themselves 'conditions', but rather the outcome of activities, which Spector and Kitsuse term 'claimsmaking' (p. 72–3). A primary task of the researcher therefore is to examine how some situation or condition is asserted to be morally objectionable, and how collective activity is organised around these definitions and assertions. As Spector and Kitsuse say, 'the central problem of a theory of social problems is to account for the emergence, nature, and maintenance of claims-making and responding activities' p. 76).

The social problem analyst is not concerned with whether or not 'condition x' even exists, let alone with whether it is in some final sense 'truly' morally objectionable. Rather, she or he must analyse the discourse on the existence of the problem as 'factual claims-making" and the moral discourse as 'value claims-making'. Factual and value claims are interwoven throughout the career of the problem, and Spector and Kitsuse propose four 'phases' in which this career can be divided:

> Stage One is that in which a group or groups point to the existence of some condition (a factual claim), indicate that it is undesirable in some way (a value claim), and attempt to promote it to a higher position on the agenda of public and political debate.

In Stage Two, some official organisation or institution recognises the 'truth' of the knowledge-claim, or at least begins an official investigation to clarify these claims, and begins to formulate an official 'policy response'.

In Stage Three the original groups declare themselves unsatisfied with official response, and the 'policy failure' or 'cover-up' becomes a new problem claim.

In Stage Four, claims-making groups abandon their attempt to satisfy their grievances and/or to resolve the asserted problem through official channels and begin to develop 'alternative' parallel, or counter-institutions'.

This 'stages model' is not put forward by Spector and Kitsuse as anything more than a working hypothesis. They do not assume that social problems have any 'natural history', let alone the specific one which they have outlined. They hope, however, that eventually:

> The original counsel of the natural history concept to examine sequences of events and to document unfolding lines of activities will have produced a rich literature ... a hypothetical natural history may serve as a temporary procedural manual, checklist of things to attend to, and a first order of business. (p. 158)

The procedure advocated by Spector and Kitsuse is to investigate the claims-making strategies of all the groups engaged in a social problem process, which may include a wide variety of profess-ions, pressure groups, 'moral crusaders', official agencies and members of the media. An essential part of this investigation is to 'ascertain how participants in an activity define that activity' (p. 79).

A critical elaboration of this approach as it can be applied to the British policy process is offered by Manning (1985). Like Spector and Kitsuse, he takes a 'developmental' approach, and focuses on the process of claims-making rather than on the questions of 'whether the problem really exists'. This is not a 'natural' but rather a 'social history'. To Spector and Kitsuse's stages he adds a possible 'loop' back from the third to the second stages (an example is the setting up of a Royal Commission) and observes that 'Group claims can get stuck in this loop and disappear' (pp. 9–10) He describes two processes which accompany the progress of social-problem claims through these stages: the 'individualisation' of social problems (which I will call 'moral fragmentation') and, following Nelkin (1975), the tendency for social problems to become defined as the exclusive territory of experts (which I will call 'technical fragmentation').

His criticism of his predecessors is that the model does not go into sufficient detail about the ways in which claims are put forward by some groups and accepted by others, nor about what determines the way 'official and government agencies react.

Manning devotes more attention than Spector and Kitsuse to the nature of 'the state'. He sees the state as a 'site of conflicts and struggle' over the allocation of goods and services. Claims upon the state for goods and services are made by pressure groups of various kinds, and here the analysis of J. J. Richardson and A. G. Jordan (1979) is a useful addition to the social problem model. Richardson and Jordan go so far as to argue that, in the course of social-problem processes, that: 'there is a breaking-down of conceptual distinctions between government, agencies and pressure groups; an interpenetration of departmental and client groups (p. 44). They contend that officials and pressure groups are to some extent symbiotic. One reason for this, which is not spelt out explicitly by Richardson and Jordan but which was spoken of by participants in the debate described here, is the need for an official wishing to carve out a 'career', to be seen to initiate and/or promote a successful programme or innovation. Contact with pressure groups and 'dissident' academics can be a good source of 'bright ideas' which, when used with skill and discretion, benefit officials' careers.

Richardson and Jordan offer their own version of the 'stages model' of a social problem process, based on that of Downs. In this model, more prominence is given (than that accorded in Spector and Kitsuse's version) to two additional 'stages':

1. The 'dramatic event' which alerts the public to the issue.
2. The 'decline of public interest' which sets in once the high cost of 'solving' the problem has been realised (p. 90)

They point out that process 2 may be 'helped along' by the promotion of new issues onto the agenda of public debate, pushing out the old (from Downs, 1973). They dismiss the idea that the policy agenda is set by pressure groups and interest groups openly lobbying the legislature; 'campaigns are the currency of unsuccessful groups; permanent relationships are the mode of the successful' (p. 123).

The reason these 'permanent relationships' are given little

prominence in the literature on policy-making is that their confi-
dentiality is one of their essential characteristics. Richardson and
Jordan admit that if the presence of a strong pressure group is
combined with parliamentary interest and good media coverage,
policy actions *can* be brought about by 'outsiders', but they feel
that this is the exception rather than the rule.

The role of the media

Manning also points out that Spector and Kitsuse have no analysis of the role of the media in the social problem process. Carole
Weiss, who has written extensively on the question of how information is used to influence policy-makers (for example, Weiss
1982), notes that:

> generalisations and ideas from numbers of studies come
> into currency ... through articles in academic journals, jour-
> nals of opinion, stories in the media ... lobbying by special
> interest groups, conversations of colleagues, attendance at
> conferences ... and other uncatalogued sources ... (p. 290)

Adopting the phrase originated by Shils (1961), she describes this
as the 'enlightenment model' of the relationship between research
and policy. Due to the important role played by the media in the
'networks of enlightenment' described by Weiss, certain important agenda-setting decisions are taken by the journalists who
control claims-making groups' access to newspaper space and
airtime. These decisions take the form of concepts of 'newsworthi-
ness' which are well described by various writers on the media
(such as Goldenberg 1975, Altheide and Johnson 1980).

Work on pressure groups and the media, such as that of Oscar
Gandy (1982), Field (1982) and Banting (1979) demonstrates that
pressure group activity often involves the making of 'knowledge-
claims' as a central concern. These authors point out that 'scientists' and 'policy actors' (both those who wish to change the status
quo and those who wish to preserve it) all make use of public
controversy, often 'creating' such debate through that form of
skilful use of the media, which Gandy describes as 'information
subsidy'. As he puts it:

> The information is characterised as a subsidy because the
> source of that information causes it to be made available at
> something less than the cost a user would face in the absence
> of a subsidy ... That is, the delivery of an information sub-
> sidy through the news media may involve an effort that

> reduces the cost of producing news faced by a reporter, journalist or editor. (pp. 61–2)

Gandy's work applies only secondarily to professional or scientific groups, but forms an extremely useful model for the more public phases of the unemployment and health debate. He points out:

> Politicians, bureaucrats, producers and consumers will each attempt to influence the identification of social problems, the formulation of policy options in response to those problems ... They will attempt to produce that influence ... most frequently through the provision of information subsidy to other policy actors. (p. 55)

Gandy points out that pressure groups and entrepreneurial subprofessions often act as 'expert' providers of subsidised information to the media in order to put pressure on political administrators ('the State'), and bring about or prevent policy change:

> Faced with time constraints, and the need to produce stories that will win publication, journalists will attend to, and make use of, subsidised information ... By reducing the costs faced by journalists in satisfying organisational requirements, the subsidy giver increases the probability that the subsidised information will be used. (p. 62)

How can interest-groups thus 'reduce the costs' to a journalist of using their information? This question was itself a recurring topic for participants in the unemployment and health debate. Activists and (a few) researchers learned how to write a press release so as to hit the right balance between presentation of qualified factual information and 'sensationalism' They strove to guess what would carry authority (one of the first things some journalists wanted to know of the provider of a subsidy was 'Is s/he a doctor?'). They discovered the value of making something appear to be a 'leak'.

Relating his discussion of pressure groups to that of the media, Manning points out that pressure groups have usually:

> developed an intimate relationship with the mass media [and that ... out of this relationship, particularly the exercise of journalistic routines ... comes an image amongst 'informed' opinion as to how grievances should be perceived and whether the resulting claims are legitimate. (p. 19)

The media alone, however, cannot create major social problems. In order for this to happen, larger 'power blocs' must become involved. These may be successful social movements, business concerns, or they may also be alliances of professional groups. Pressure groups on single issues must, therefore, gain the support of these wider constituencies. A social-problem analysis needs to describe the ways in which small pressure groups seek to have their claims taken up by more powerful bodies.

Scientific claims-making

One fairly common way of strengthening claims is to make appeals to 'science'. Up to the present, few researchers within the social problems perspective have pursued their topics very far into the laboratory or research institute, although claims about scientific truth appear with great frequency in social problem processes. A rare example of an approach combining insights from social-problems theory and the sociology of scientific knowledge is Aronson's account of nutrition policy in early twentieth century America. Aronson (1982a) shows how a long drawn-out effort by Atwater, the leading entrepreneurial figure in the new subdiscipline of nutrition science, produced 'dietary ignorance' as a concept. The new concept served to mediate between the concerns of a new science struggling for recognition and funding, the US government, and American labour reformers wishing to improve the lot of the industrial worker and quell civil unrest without changing basic economic structures. Labour movement agitation during the period 1870–80), concerned with the inadequacy of wages, provided the occasion for the scientists to claim to 'have the answer'. By fragmenting the 'labour problem' into a technical question of measuring nutritional sufficiency, and a moral one of educating the poor in correct dietary practices, they were able to offer the conclusion that existing wage levels were sufficient if correct dietary principles were observed. In this way, a 'political' problem concerning the adequacy of wages became a 'social problem' concerning dietary ignorance. As part of the same process Atwater and his followers established their knowledge claims as important 'facts' for use in the policy-making process.

At present the sociology of science has begun to give more prominence to the social and economic context of scientific work, partly as a result of the growing consensus that change in scientific ideas cannot be understood as the simple pursuit of accurate accounts of an 'external reality'. Work in the sociology of scientific knowledge (SSK) has shown that closure of a scientific debate can never be regarded as the result of discoveries about a world 'out there' because there is simply no such thing as a universally acceptable 'replication' of any scientific experiment (Collins 1983, 1985). Therefore, closure of debate, and the outcome of closure known as 'discovery of a fact' must be studied as social processes. An important contribution to understanding these processes is provided by the 'interest model' developed by (amongst others) Barnes (1977), Bloor (1976) and Mackenzie (1981a).

There have now been many case studies using some variation of an 'interest model' to investigate scientific debates, and the empirical study of scientists at work (whether or not they were engaged in public controversy) has led to a rich elaboration of this model which increases its usefulness to the study of policy-related scientific controversies. Some of these have been micro-level studies of scientists at work in the 'laboratory'; situation (the term 'laboratory' will be used here, as it is in the work quoted, to mean any working situation in which scientists are found, whether or not it contains the accoutrements we would normally think of). Foremost among these both in its relevance to field material and perhaps also in the general estimation, is Latour and Woolgar's (1979, 1986) 'Laboratory Life'.

In their close observation of scientists at work, Latour and Woolgar developed the concept of the 'cycle of credibility'. They give this name to what might be regarded as the typical or 'normal' career strategy of a scientist, whereby he or she 'invests' time and skills according to a calculation of the best achievable outcome. Such calculation is regarded by scientists as a necessary part of the exercise of their profession, and success in certain individuals is attributed to an inspired ability to make correct investment decisions. The outcome of these decisions, in the form of published papers, invitations to address conferences, and other signs of approval and acceptance, in turn attract resources such as new grants, valued colleagues, additional equipment. This enables the scientist to increase her next investment, with a correspondingly expected increase in returns, and so on. Knorr-Cetina (1982) has commented on the phenomenon:

> Scientists talk about their 'investments' in an area of research, or an experiment. They are aware of the 'risks', 'costs' and 'returns' connected with their efforts, and talk of 'selling' their results to particular journals or foundations.

This analysis of the ways in which individual academic scientists' and research groups' agendas are formed points us even more firmly in the direction of the wider social-problem processes which constitute the context of scientific work.

This approach is both criticised and elaborated by Knorr-Cetina (1982). She disagrees with the 'quasi-economic' concept of investment and return on the grounds that when limited to the interior of science, these concepts have insufficient explanatory power. The decisions made in the laboratory appear to be simultaneously situated in a field of social relations (p. 102). This is the 'trans-scientific field', which is 'organised in terms of resource-relationships' ... the transepistemic connections of research are *built into* scientific inquiry'. Knorr-Cetina criticises Latour and Woolgar for not taking account of the relations between scientific producers and their clients in the creation of 'true accounts' of phenomena. She warns against equating the sort of conditionally accepted 'information' (knowledge claims) which scientists strive to produce in order to gain recognition by their peers *within* the scientific community with a wider concept of 'truth'. In order for a 'truth' to be established, a further step is required, and this she sees as the intervention of *entrepreneurs*. And it is not only the final step in the fact-creating process (from 'information' to 'truth') which requires entrepreneurship. Knorr-Cetina also reminds us that science is 'a system in which a scientist's ability to work, including the ability to raise money, may depend on decisions made at the top organisational and other administrative levels (p. 112).

And at *these* levels, the scientific cycle of credibility plays no part in the making of decisions, she argues. At this level, questions of allocating resources are paramount. The present study will not exactly follow Knorr-Cetina here:what seems to happen at the level at which resource decisions are taken (funding bodies, government departments), as far as this can be ascertained, is that certain individuals or subgroups may take up a research team' s case and push it as a part of their *own* cycle of credibility. The impression given by Knorr-Cetina that somehow there are 'big decisions' about resources taken in a different manner from those about 'facts' is at least partly an artefact of difficulties of research access to decision-making sites. It is important that this practical question of fieldwork method and strategy not be allowed to construct a monolith at the level of 'the state'.

Knorr-Cetina does warn of the dangers of merely *assuming* the relationship between 'credibility' and resources. Should we take it ₁or granted that a scientist who is accorded much credibility (through the reception of his or her published work, as 'true' 'excellent', etc.) by peers will be more likely to receive further resources to invest in the next phase of the cycle? Knorr-Cetina thinks not, and this forms another of her criticisms of Latour and Woolgar's concentration on the inside of the laboratory. Other laboratory studies have shown the scientists deemed 'successful' in this sense have been deprived of their funds and equipment in what seems to them a completely arbitrary manner, or, conversely, find that previously rejected proposals suddenly find favour in the eyes of those who control access to resources. Although scientists retain partial control of their own time, they are nevertheless still primarily *workers* in 'a market of positions where the commodity is scientists' (Knorr-Cetina 1982, p. 112) who must 'sell their labour power' like any other worker. Here we can see that Knorr-Cetina is not really objecting to the 'quasi-economic model' of science, but to an inconsistent or incomplete model which fails to distinguish the role of 'worker' from that of 'entrepreneur' and 'employer'. An individual scientist may, at various times, behave as if s/he were any one of these (giving rise to such descriptions of academic activity as 'time-serving', 'getting on a bandwagon', and 'empire-building', respectively). But Knorr-Cetina aims at greater conceptual clarity when analysing the process of scientific investigation, and holds that such clarity will take us outside the laboratory.

Indeed, the concept of a community of knowledge-producers as one composed solely or even mainly of scientists is not accurate. Although this study has made some use of a concept of 'the core group' (Collins 1981) of researchers who remained longest involved in the centre of the unemployment and health debate, this group included non-researchers. Nor is a picture of a self-contained group of scientists provided by an ethnographic description of what scientists do (Pinch and Bijker 1984). In Knorr-Cetina's's fieldwork, as in the present study, the scientists themselves do not orient solely or even mainly towards each other, depending on the stage at which the process of debate is observed. Much of Knorr-Cetina's criticism of laboratory studies implies the importance of a missing *temporal* dimension, and it was the longitudinal character of the present study which demanded the addition of a social-problem perspective to concepts drawn purely from the laboratory micro-studies, useful as these were in understanding much interview material. In the course of close ethnographic observation:

> We see scientists writing letters and sending out papers and grant proposals. We hear them talking to people all over the country on the phone ... We read the correspondence filed away in a folder and learn about contracts realised for industry ... we learn that they *frame* their scientific work in terms of their ex situ involvements. (Knorr-Cetina 1982, p. 117)

Furthermore, these negotiations are woven tightly into what will ultimately result as a knowledge claim. The network of relationships in which the scientist is involved thus enters fully into the resulting 'facts' Knorr-Cetina does not regard this network as directly observable. In the present case study, an attempt has been made to observe a large part of such a network, tracing those connections perceived as significant by scientific (and other) participants by means of reading the documents and correspondence produced and referred to, and by interviewing members of the groups making up the 'trans-scientific' field for the academic debate.

We are left, still, with the problem of finding an alternative to the mere assumption that 'credibility' is automatically translated into resources. When scientists reach out along their networks seeking for resources, what do they offer in return, what are they 'selling'? Knorr-Cetina suggests that it is 'the convertibility of ... a scientist's work into the locally relevant "currencies"' (p. 121). That is, we cannot even assume anything about what may *count* as a resource, either sought for or offered in return by the scientists in their wider relationships. It may be money or equipment or space or time. It may be legitimation. The fragility of the definition of a 'resource' is reflected in the amount of effort put into writing research proposals, she argues. Furthermore, and here again the social-problem perspective is a good guide, scientists may seek to convert what they already have (a new statistical measure for example, or a medical procedure, or a 'unique' set of data) into a resource relevant to some other group's own aims. What this means is that the analyst cannot be too quick to make simple assumptions about what will be sought for or offered as a resource. Rather, it is necessary to listen to what subjects say. As it was observed in the unemployment and health debate, so also in Knorr-Cetina's study, 'oscillations between conflict and co-opera-

tion, between the fission and fusion of interests that are recipro-
cally defined, are routine correlates of the process of negotiation
which characterizes resource-relationships' (1982, p. 122).

Accordingly, the analyst must not assume that somehow 'society'
provides an input into science in the form of setting social problems for science to solve. Scientists are not passive recipients of
either resources or 'questions', but rather active participants in
the social-problem process through which 'problems' are defined.
Social and political issues may reach deeply into the design and
analysis of research. But equally, available and/or well-marketed
scientific skills and techniques will influence what comes to be
solidified as a 'researchable issue'. Furthermore, scientists (and
policy-makers, and research funders inside and outside of government) must always be to some extent engaged in a process of
striving for or approximating a desired relationship between concerns deriving from the trans-scientific field (the social, medical,
etc., 'problems' at stake) and the design of measures, tests, samples, and other 'laboratory' procedures. Even when there appears
to be complete agreement between customers and contractors:

> Scientists 'figure', 'gather', 'think' and 'hope' that a particu-
> lar problem translation ... will match the interest of those
> to whom they are committed, but they often do not *know*
> *exactly* what is expected from them. So they re-direct their
> guesswork according to the responses they get, and they
> may end up convincing those who are 'interested' in the
> work about what exactly they should be interested in.
> (Knorr-Cetina 1982, p. 124)

Out of this negotiating, guessing and figuring not only about the
natural world but also about the characteristics of the research
team's *social* world which need to be correctly managed in order
to advance the (individual and collective) aims of team members,
emerge 'facts' and 'knowledge'.

The organisation of science and the social-problem process

The most recent and sophisticated work on the process of 'translation' between scientists' concerns and those of significant groups
in the 'trans-scientific' field comes from France (Callon 1981, 1986;
Law and Rip 1986; Latour 1984a, b; Coutouzis and Latour 1986;
Latour 1987). An account of the theoretical and methodological
bases upon which this research is constructed shows the close
relationship between a translation programme for the sociology

of scientific knowledge and the social problems perspective.

Callon and Law (1982) see the 'networking' activities of scientists as 'an attempt to determine the relative "marketability" of different fields of work', for example, in choosing what questions to pursue, selecting the journals to which they will send papers, the funding bodies to whom they will appeal, and so on. All these activities involve attempts to first 'interest' (this term now being used with the specific meaning of 'actively attract the interest of') and then 'enrol' others in the scientists' own projects. As Callan and Law (1982) put it: 'Analytically, [the scientists'] position is little different from a politician who uses argument and persuasion to insist that it is in the 'interests' of this or that social group to vote in this or that way' (square brackets are author's).

For these researchers 'interesting' ('interessement') is an activity in which scientists engage, for example, when they target a paper at a specific journal or a grant application at a particular funding body (Law 1983). Furthermore, their concept of enrolment is not unidirectional. If a researcher 'sells' a paper to a journal, s/he has enrolled the journal in his or her scheme of things. If the editors ask for major changes and get them, however, then it is the scientist who has been 'enrolled'. The question of 'interests', for Callon and Law, is therefore 'to discover how it is that actors enrol one another, and why it is that some succeed whereas others do not.' One strategy of enrolment, as illustrated by Knorr-Cetina, is to guess what the interests of others are, and adapt one's work accordingly.

This working-through of the consequences of regarding science as a thoroughly social activity leads back towards the social-problems model, and to the ways in which an integration of the two approaches can enable steps forward to be taken in the understanding of policy-related scientific debates. A sociology of scientific knowledge which places scientists so firmly as active subjects within a social world in which they participate as knowledgeable, artful and striving to attain certain personal and group objectives seems to fit well with a programme to treat social problems as organised phenomena with their own variable 'social histories'. As Latour (1981, 1987) insists, there is nothing sacred or special about science. It is a social activity amongst others. So it should not come as a surprise that concepts found useful in the analysis of scientists' activities, in the present study, proved applicable, with some modification, to understanding the activities of members of other groups in the 'issue community'. Latour (1987, p. 168) advocates that in studying the fate of scientific ideas, 'we should not consider only those who called themselves scientists – the tip of the iceberg – but those who, although they stay outside, are nevertheless shaping the science, and form the bulk of the iceberg'. This is necessary because 'scientists ... link their fate to that of other and much more powerful groups ... that have learned how to interest everyone in some issues ... groups that are constantly on the look-out for new unsuspected allies' (p. 169). The scientists entered the social-problem process in the same way as other groups, indeed, the conduct of the academic debate only began to become comprehensible when scientists' activities *were* theoretically approached in this way.

The Strong Programme, by opening up all forms of scientific and technical activity to sociological analysis, allows us to see that scientists are like any other participants in organised activity who compete for material and cultural resources. They make claims in relation to other scientists, and also in relation to the wider society. Just as social problems arise from the ongoing and related activities of social movements, professions, officials and journalists, so 'scientific facts' arise from the ongoing activity of scientists *in relation* to these other groups. At certain times, scientists of one sort or another are 'mobilised' by other actors in social-problem processes, to produce factual claims consistent with these actors' objectives and/or value orientations (see Harwood 1979, 1980, 1982; Gillespie, Eva and Johnston 1979; Nowotny and Hirsch 1980). At other times, scientists themselves will enter a social-problem process, or even create one, in order to advance the claims to status and resources of the research team, laboratory, or other group or institution to which they belong (as in Aronson 1982a and b). Scientists enter the fields of social-problem debate 'spontaneously' when a group of them can see that the debate offers opportunities for new and desirable alliances, that is, for mobilising others in pursuit of the scientists' own objectives. If these objectives can be attained by alternative means, then participation in any given debate or social-problem process will come to be seen as of only passing relevance.

In Latour's formulation, chains of reasoning which scientists construct forge the links of social alliances. Logic and social strategy are one and the same. A 'fact' will be established when a group of scientists establishes their argument (or artefact) as a common element which links together (perhaps provisionally and fleetingly) the majority of other groups involved in a given social-problem process. This he terms the establishment of an 'obligatory point of passage'. For example, the success of germ theory in nineteenth-century France was that its protagonists eventually established the 'microbe' as the common element to all the varied mass of phenomena (both 'biological' and 'political') with which a far greater and older social movement ('Public Health') was concerned, thus mobilising a strong ally (Latour 1984a, pp. 25–35).

From this account of the translation model of scientific controversy, we can clearly see its close similarities to a social-problem model of policy debate. In effect, Latour, Callon and their colleagues have demonstrated that the construction of fact and artefact and debates over questions of policy are inextricable. If the researcher adopts the ethnographic method advocated by the 'laboratory studies', and persistently follows or 'shadows' (in Latour's terms) the scientists in their daily work, it can be seen that an essential part of the activity of senior scientists entails discussions and negotiations with a wide variety of decision-makers outside the scientific community. Similarly, in studies of policy debate, activists and officials will be found to engage routinely in activities to enrol support on the basis of factual claims.

What emerges is a series of stages in a debate. Once groups do enter the process, they engage in:

1. Attempts to 'interest' other groups – whether these be conceptualised as 'social' (funding bodies, other professional groups, political parties) or as 'natural' [microbes, as in Latour (1984a), shellfish, as in Callon (1986), tides, as in Law (1986b].

   Here 'inter-esting' ('coming between') is taken to mean persuading a group's members to take a different course, to take a diversion down the road which the scientists (or other would-be 'inter-estors') propose. It is achieved by a form of bargaining or compromise between the ongoing activities and obectives of the scientists and those of the potential allies. The process of 'interesting' entails.

2. 'Translation', that is, mutual adjustment of the groups' ongoing activities so that they become 'resources' for each other (see Knorr-Cetina's discussion of the ways in which items may be constructed as 'resource' above).

If translation is successful, groups have succeeded in

3. 'enrolment' – the creation of a (relatively) stable set of alliances. Out of this 'lash-up' (Latour 1987) of forces emerges an *obligatory point of passage*. That is the statement or instrument which all groups accept as essential to their several purposes, the expression of the point where their 'interests' meet.

The translation school draws a close analogy between scientific debates and either political or military battles, in which all parties are engaged in seeking better ground, better weapons and stronger allies. All parties are guided in their actions by conscious strategies (and not driven by forces arising from either the mind or the social structure of which they are unaware). Outcomes are often not what was intended, but this is because, as with all social activity, the combined effect of several intentions is often a set of 'unintended consequences'.

In Part One therefore, the events described and the discussion about these events reported have been selected in the light of this model. The debate is roughly organised into a series of 'stages'. Interactions between scientists, pressure groups and policy makers are highlighted. Examples are given of the production of 'information subsidy' offered to the media, and note is taken of who offered subsidy. Attempts to forge alliances are recounted, as are the breakup of such alliances. It is fortunate that a universally accepted version of 'the effect of unemployment on health' was never reached. This removes the strong temptation to write a 'Whiggish' history of the debate which begins from an accepted truth and works backward to tell a story of error overcome. My own belief will be clear enough: that in the course of the debate a major advance was made in social statistics which potentially throws new light on the effects on health not only of unemployment but also of other forms of social inequality. But at the time of writing that is only a matter of opinion. Many others would share my sentiment that the new ideas 'have not been fully tested', and agree that they have not been widely applied. The social conditions are not fulfilled in which social and medical statisticians would generally agree that a new 'fact' has been added to the stock at their disposal. This also means there is no temptation to adopt a unidirectional model of the relationship between research and policy, and makes it easier for the following account to consider whether it may be more fruitful to concentrate on the interactive nature of this relationship.

2

'UNCOVERING THE SOCIAL PROBLEM'

The year 1974 saw a major upheaval in the organisation of the British National Health Service. One aspect of the reorganisation was a fundamental change in the role of public health, and in the status of the public health physicians, the Medical Officers of Health (MOsH). New Regional, Area and District Health Authorities took over the functions previously carrried out by Medical Officers of Health in local government Public Health Departments. The functions of the MOsH were combined with those of the Medical Administrators of the old Regional Hospital Boards, and the medical staff of the university departments of public health and social medicine, to form the new speciality of Community Medicine. The function of these specialists was to investigate and assess the needs of the population so that priorities could be established for the promotion of health and the prevention of disease, as well as the provision of medical care.

In 1975 a small research and policy unit, the Unit for the Study of Health Policy (USHP) began to operate within Guy's Hospital's Department of Community Medicine with a brief 'to promote informed discussion on health policy' at this time of change. The unit was initially funded for five years by the King Edward Hospital Fund for London ('The King's Fund'). The Unit's director was Dr Peter Draper, previously Senior Lecturer in Social Medicine at Guy's.

In December 1975, Draper read an article in *The Financial Times*, written by C. Gordon Tether who was at that time the 'Lombard' columnist. The topic was the work of an American academic, M. Harvey Brenner, on the social and health costs of unemployment. Brenner had written a report 'Estimating the social costs of national economic policy' for the US Congress Joint Economic Committee in 1976, claiming that economic policy-makers needed to take account in the unemployment rate. The article struck a chord with Draper and some of his staff in two ways. As part of their work on prevention of illness they had developed an interest in research on stress, a topic which Draper felt had tended to be neglected. The second attraction of Brenner's work was that it raised questions about whether the economic environment might have an effect on health. These interests were strong enough for Unit staff to consider organising a conference on the effects of economic change on health despite the fact that they saw unemployment as 'right off our main line' as a health policy unit.

Draper's colleague John Dennis recalled that inflation rather than unemployment was seen as the major political and economic 'problem' at that time, in wider political debate. However during the following year public concern about unemployment continued to increase as the figures continued to deteriorate. In August 1976, the number of unemployed persons in the UK was the highest total for that month since 1938: 1.5 million, or 6.4 per cent. (*The Lancet*, editorial 22 January 1977, p. 182). The Unit's workshop on the consequences of unemployment took place in Abergavenny in January 1977, entitled 'Health unemployment and ingenuity'. It was a gratifying recognition of their efforts that a member of the editorial staff of the prestigious medical journal *The Lancet* attended. *The Lancet* editorial which followed was couched in sympathetic terms:

> The direct health implications of being unemployed are many and obvious: despite the various benefits that are payable, poverty and its concomitants – bad housing, poor nutrition, sickness, and social deprivation – remain disproportionately common amongst those who are out of work. (22 January 1977, p. 182)

Despite the marginality of unemployment and its possible effect on health to the concerns of USHP, the group continued to promote Brenner's work in the UK. Their ability to do so was greatly helped by the arrival of medical students doing 'elective periods' of study in public health medicine, first Nick Joyner and later Nigel Konzon, who both wrote high quality literature reviews on unemployment and health as their project work. Joyner and a fellow student in the same year, Stephen Wood were among the organisers of a series of meetings on 'issues in health care' aimed at broadening the perspective of medical students at Guys. In November 1977, Wood invited Prof Peter Townsend to speak to the 'Issues in Health Care' group. After the meeting, Wood wrote to Townsend:

It is all too infrequent that medical students have the opportunity to hear about such important topics as poverty and
unemployment [although] – I am optimistic (or perhaps
naive) enough to hope that the ostrich-like attitude to social
and economic questions so predominant in medicine may
be on its way out.

He enclosed with the letter a copy of Joyner's project paper. As a
result, Townsend referred Nick Joyner to his colleague at Essex
University, Adrian Sinfield, who had carried out one of the few
existing sociological studies of unemployed people in post-war
Britain, for advice. However, it is the nature of student electives
that, although they may inspire considerable effort and be of good
quality, they are then 'left behind' as the student faces his or her
final year of study and examinations. Neither Wood nor Joyner
(who both went on to study and practice psychiatry) nor Konzon
(who later took over a general practice in Brixton's 'front line'
area) ever took up the issue of unemployment again, although
their actions produced the first signals between the medical and
social policy worlds that there was some medical interest in unemployment.

Another speaker at an 'Issues in Health Care' group in 1977
was Dr Len Fagin, a psychiatrist whose undergraduate medical
training in Argentina gave him a perspective on community
health issues which was particularly interesting to the group. His
talk dealt with the effect of unemployment on the mental and
physical health of families. Having studied with the acknowledged British expert on bereavement, Murray Parkes, he had an
interest in reactions to loss and the conditions which aided or
hindered the recuperative powers of the individual. The problem
with unemployment, he argued, was that people were not
supposed to learn to accept it and 'recover' from the experience of
loss. This, to his mind, produced the risk of prolonged stress, and
he wished to investigate the effects on physical as well as mental
health.

Like the three students and several USHP staff, Fagin was an
occasional attender of meetings of a new discussion group, the
Politics of Health Group (POHG) which began to meet during
1977. As he put it, coming from Buenos Aires had engendered 'a
concern with the connection between political and economic
events and health.' Practising as a psychiatrist in the East End of
London confirmed these sympathies, and provided him with

plenty of clinical examples in the form of patients who were unemployed. During this year, Fagin initiated a research project which which received a great deal of media and parliamentary attention.

Fagin and his colleague Martin Little, a psychiatric social worker, had approached the Manpower Services Commission (MSC) to see whether they could study a factory closure. Objections from both management and unions proved too strong a barrier: 'People just were not interested in talking to researchers in 1977. The unions thought we were on the management's side and the management thought we were on the unions' side.'

They tried various other methods for picking up a sample of unemployed people – standing outside benefit offices, going through GPs' lists and social services departments' referrals. None were successful. They then heard 'through the grapevine' about a longitudinal study of unemployed men being carried out by researchers in the Department of Health and Social Security (the DHSS Cohort Study). As Fagin remember: 'They were interested because they realised it was going to be a bit of a superficial statistical exercise, and it might be a useful adjunct to have a small descriptive survey attached to it.'

The DHSS researchers agreed to contact a sub-sample of Cohort Study (CS) families to see if they were willing to be interviewed by Fagin and Little. Access to families now settled, they faced the problem of getting funding. First they approached the MSC who turned down their proposal: 'they said they didn't think they'd get a lot of return from a psychological study at this stage.' They then approached the local health research group who felt that the proposal was 'not worked out enough.' Eventually, after more work, the proposal was submitted through the DHSS's Small Grant Scheme, and was awarded £2,400 over two years.

Len Fagin was a registrar at this time, and, in common with registrars in many other medical sub-specialties, would have been not only permitted but expected to carry out research as part of the preparation for the post of consultant. Accordingly, he used his study time to carry out the interviews. They interviewed twenty-two families chosen to be representative of the CS sample.

The resulting report (Fagin 1981), which was a largely qualitative account of the families' experiences of and reactions to unemployment, was then presented to their sponsors in the winter of 1981. The report and its reception by the media and in Parliament will be discussed further below, but in the interim period, a series of events had changed the tone of the debate.

The Reckoning

In November 1978, Harvey Brenner was invited to speak at Guy's Hospital for the first time, at a meeting organised by USHP. In the meantime, his work had also come to the attention of Granada Television's 'World in Action' team. USHP staff did not remember whether this had happened through them or not. Granada asked Brenner to study two areas felt to be contrasting in terms of unemployment levels at that time, Nottingham and Liverpool. Some USHP staff were left with the impression that the producer and the programme's researcher had suffered a certain amount of interference in their attempts to promote and realise the idea, that moves had been made to prevent it being shown, and that the fact that it was not billed in *TV Times* or the daily papers' TV guides was an attempt to minimise its impact. For example on 12 February 1979 Peter Draper wrote to Brenner:

> We ... half suspect a Machiavellian plot to minimise interest once the powers that be decide they couldn't actually *kill* the programme (too many people knew of its existence) ... I think it is most important that the Community Medicine establishment and the DHSS aren't allowed to get away with simply dismissing your work.

And a USHP staff member 'couldn't decide what the truth of it was. I veered between thinking I was being either paranoid or naive'. However, a Granada journalist expressed shock at these suspicions:

> It is greatly to Granada's credit (he felt) that they do not interfere too much with how the programme is made ... What we make depends entirely on those twenty-four people (the World in Action team of researchers and producers). If you work for the programme, you put up your ideas ... It's not just a question of having a bright idea, you have to fight for it. ... TV ... is an accident-prone process. There are no conspiracies involved in the making of documentary programmes ... Half our programmes are not billed in *TV Times* because no-one knows which one is going to be finished on time.

The same journalist related on a separate occasion that Brenner had had to be filmed twice, at great expense to Granada, because of the importance given to getting the interview right: 'It was the longest interview we've ever done on World in Action.' And a USHP worker admitted; 'it had problems, it was what I call statistical television. The figures for deaths sort of sprang out of the screen at you.'

News of the programme's progress reached the attention of some Labour MPs even before it was screened. On 23 January 1979 Mr Geoff Rooker asked in a Parliamentary Question (PQ) whether the Minister for Health would 'institute an inquiry into the relationship between unemployment and illness, so that his Department is not stimulated to take that action following a forthcoming Granada Television programme?' Mr Albert Booth replied rather limply:

> I see it as part of the role of my Department, working with the Health and Safety Executive, to watch carefully the relationship between unemployment and illness, and to take steps to institute good health and safety practices to avoid loss of employment in that way

thus genuinely or wilfully misunderstanding the point of the question.

The Reckoning was shown on 5 February 1979. On the day of the screening, alerted by a 'World in Action' researcher, USHP members attempted to overcome the absence of any billing in the newspapers by phoning interested parties to tell them the programme was on, and also by taping it. One USHP staff member related its impact:

> The House of Commons requested a copy and then there was a lot of interest. USHP got phone calls from civil servants asking where they could get copies of the Senate report [a reference to Brenner's report to the Joint Economic Committee of the US Congress]. We organised a small technical seminar which Harvey gave. The focus was on Harvey's model ... [Some] people were concerned with the techniques. There were civil servants there too. One main reason for setting up the workshop was because of the interest shown by policy-makers. We kept getting phone calls from civil servants.

Present at the seminar were several people from the professional research staff of the DHSS. One of these explained their presence in the following way:

> The DHSS were interested in knowing what the costs of the

rising rate of unemployment were going to be as far as they were concerned. At this time the Labour party were in power and they were also worried about it. So for the time being the interests of officials and politicians were more or less the same.

Further linking the subject to health service allocation, a topical issue at the time, he went on:

The second reason they were interested in whether what Brenner was saying had anything in it was because of health service planning needs. In trying to allocate resources between areas, you are always looking for indicators. If there was anything in this unemployment/health business, it might mean that either an increased demand might arise, or it might be useful as an indicator for allocation of services and local health authority provision. Did it mean we needed some sort of monitoring system?

And another powerful source of civil service interest was invoked:

The third thing was a Whitehall point. You see, departments are always looking for the best way of presenting their expenditure claims. At the time there was a lot of emphasis on Special Employment Measures and Job Creation ... So the question arose, to what extent should we be using the long term unemployed in jobs like unskilled work in the health service? Whenever a government department puts in expenditure claims, the Treasury resists them. Relating unemployment to special measures was a way of legitimating claims ... The key issue as far as Brenner was concerned, for the Department, was, 'here's all this song and dance – what work do *we* need to commission in the light of it?' Both officials and Ministers wanted to know.

USHP therefore succeeded in attracting the attention of government advisers and officials, even before the first academic publication of their ideas on unemployment and health. Further Parliamentary Questions followed. Shortly after the screening of *The Reckoning* Mr Rooker wrote to Undersecretary of State for Labour, John Golding, expressing disquiet at the Labour Party's position on possible health risks of unemployment. The answer to this letter indicates the defensiveness of government ministers of any colour in the face of politically sensitive research. On 1 March Golding replied:

Although there is an association between unemployment
and ill-health, it is difficult to prove that unemployment is itself
a cause ... since unemployment is often a consequence of poor
health, accidents or prolonged illness [here a note scribbled
on the margin of the letter exclaims 'with 1.4 million!'].
Some researchers have deduced, from much the same statistics as Professor Brenner, that employment, rather than unemployment, is the most important determin-ant of ill-
health and mortality. There are also problems in proving
that unemployment rather than poverty causes ill-health,
since the factors are all interrelated. These questions are
being explored in the DHSS's research programme, and to
some extent also in the Department of Employment's research on the social costs of unemployment.

The information provided in both answers to Mr Rooker will
have been provided by professional civil service research officers,
and demonstrate a considerable awareness of the research. It is
considerably better-informed, for example, than subsequent interventions in the unemployment and health debate by Labour
MPs after the party left office and lost the services of these officials.[1]

The reference to the dangers of work could have been a reference to the deliberations of the DHSS working group on inequalities in health (published in 1980 and widely known as 'The Black
Report'). Or it could have been to an academic debate which had
taken place in 1977 in the pages of the *International Journal of
Health Services* between Brenner and the leading American antagonist of his work, Joseph Eyer (who could be considered politically far to the left of Brenner). Here, as is often the case, 'backstage' civil servants were intellectually on top of the issues raised
by MPs, and in a position to outbid anything seen as left-wing
pressure whether from outside the governing party or within it.

In *The Lancet* of 17 February 1979 Peter Draper's team published
the first British academic paper in the post-war unemployment
and health debate, entitled 'Micro-processors, macro-economic
policy, and public health'. The key finding of Brenner's work
(they wrote) was that a one per cent increase in the unemployment rate in the United States sustained over a period of six years
'has been associated ... with increases of approximately 36,887
total deaths' (*The Lancet*, 1979, 17 Febuary, p. 373). They advocated, as a policy response 'a transfer of funds from the social

security side of the DHSS to the health side.' These funds would be used to employ jobless people in the health service.

A 'manifesto' for public health

On 31 March 1979 a leading article 'Does unemployment kill?' was published in *The Lancet*, once again signalling recognition of the importance of the issue within the wider medical profession. It reminds readers that unemployment has now reached what its editorial staff regarded as an unprecedented post-war level of 5 per cent, and comments: 'If [Brenner's] theory is correct then the rising unemployment rate in Britain ought by now to have been associated with mortality considerable enough to put the nation's economy firmly in the domain of community health.'

This leader echoes the statistic that had been found so 'media-presentable' by 'World in Action', that 'a 1 per cent rise in unemployment sustained over a six year period could bring about 36,890 deaths in the United States,' and adds: 'If unemployment is indeed the new 'great plague', then perhaps we should call up the shades of Chadwick and his peers and make a public health attack with all the missionary zeal and authoritarianism of the nineteenth century.'

These references to the shades of Chadwick and 'missionary zeal' would have been music to the ears of the USHP (and may have been written by one or more of them). The ideas on health policy propounded by Peter Draper and his staff were part of a wider movement of opinion within public health ('community') medicine. A major theme in the work of the Unit was the need to return public health back to the centre of the political agenda, as it had been in the mid-nineteenth century when great reformers such as Chadwick had persuaded central and local governments to build the sanitary infrastructure of towns and cities. During 1978 and 1979, USHP staff and sympathisers with their work outside the Unit were also taking part in an attempt to give their ideas about the importance of the relationship between health and economic policy a more organised expression. A series of informal group discussions at the annual conference of the professional organisation of public health doctors, the Faculty of Community Medicine in June of 1978 had led to a circular being sent round by a Specialist in Information and Planning (a public health specialist) from Liverpool health authority, Alex Scott-Samuel. The letter proposed that a regular discussion group be formed.

The interested group comprised five trainees in community medicine and six academics, with only three fully qualified consultants or 'Specialists in Community Medicine' (SCMs) being included. They met in late November, and drew up a 'manifesto' of their own, highlighting such issues as

- Can community physicians be apolitical?
- Are data value-free?
- Should health services be under local political control?
- Can we accept a cut-price National Health Service. (At this time, Labour was still in power it should be remembered.)

In January of 1979 there were twenty-eight signatories (including Peter Draper) to a letter, entitled 'Radical community medicine', which was sent to the editor of the journal, *Community Medicine*, and duly published. In the same edition of the journal, an article by Scott-Samuel on 'The politics of health' was also published, which must have added to the impact of the letter. Early in March, a meeting was held between some of the signatories (who had all been doctors) and non-medical members of another small pressure group, the Radical Statistics Group, which included young statisticians trained in and committed to the ideas around 'social indicators'. What all had in common was a commitment to the importance of research on population topics as a guide to policy decisions. This group proposed the publication of 'a ten-page newsletter, say quarterly'. They called it *Radical Community Medicine*, which soon grew into a small journal. Scott-Samuel took on the role of 'catalyst' (as he saw it) or co-ordinator, on a temporary basis, a role which was to continue for five years. The statisticians demurred from what they saw as a 'medical-dominated' orientation of the newsletter, although friendly contact continued between the two groups.

Beating the government over the head

In May 1979, a General Election swept a new Conservative government into power with a large majority. This did produce some change in the ways in which certain participants dealt with the debate on unemployment and health – participants who were actively identified with the Labour party no longer had to take care not to 'embarrass ministers'.[2] It began to be seen as an unqualified advantage if research on unemployment and health produced 'something to beat the government over the head with', in the words of a member of USHP's staff. From now on, for example, questions to ministers were more likely to be put openly from the floor of the House of Commons rather than in letters to be dealt with as 'Private Office cases'. On the other hand, although dissent from government policies could be made more openly, supporting research was made more problematic. Restrictions on the funding of university research meant that members of 'expert' disciplines had to be both more careful and more entrepreneurial in the contests for research funding. Certain sorts of claims, which might have embarrassed a social-democratic administration into action (or at least into 'research') would increasingly be found to fall upon deaf ears.

The USHP suffered a setback at this point. Its Kings Fund money came to an end, and it was forced to fall back on temporary funding from the Charities Aid Foundation. The group did not publish any further papers in academic journals on unemployment and health. According to Unit staff, unemployment and health had never been a central project. One felt that:'after [the 1979 paper] came out ... we had played our role as a policy group, It was on the agenda now.'

It was not so much the priority given the issue by USHP, but the expertise of Peter Draper's team in interesting wider groups in public health topics, which made them the 'entrepreneurs' of this social problem. Peter Draper remembered that:

> We felt very lonely suggesting links between the economy and public health in those days; the 'causal' experts, the epidemiologists, seemed to be silent on such matters. Nowadays [1987] ... it all seems so obvious, but it felt quite different then! Unemployment and health felt as though it was something of a research indulgence rather than basic territory.

Mortality and economy

Brenner's own paper 'Mortality and the national economy – A review, and the experience of England and Wales, 1936–1976' was published in *The Lancet* on 15 September 1979. Draper and his colleagues remembered having 'pressed' Brenner to write the paper. The headline content of the paper was derived from its conclusion, using a complicated econometric model, that unemployment led to rises in mortality rates. In the light of the role Brenner's ideas were to play in subsequent events and argument, it is interesting to re-examine some of what he actually said in this first publication in a British academic journal. His approach is Keynesian, exemplified in the following:

> Long-term economic growth will also moderate the problems associated with economic instability: management of the national economy improves, health care gets better in quality and availability, and more substantial income support can be provided for displaced workers and other non-participants in the labour force. (p. 573)

There is an underlying theme in his work, not just in this paper, that economic management can and should be used to moderate health consequences of inevitable technological change.

One of the most controversial aspects of the paper was that the 'extra deaths' appeared to take place some time after the peak in unemployment. The reason Brenner gives for the long and diverse 'lag periods' in his model are both medical and sociological. Not only are today's 'killer diseases' chronic ones such as coronary heart disease, stroke and cancer (in contrast to the nineteenth-century plagues of acute infections), but Brenner is quite clear that recession's health-related effects upon those still in the workforce include the effects of work stress, downgrading and reintegration, as well as joblessness:

> In this sequence of 'downward social mobility' the illness process begins with recession, and, within two or three years, the likelihood of mortality is greatly increased ... For the downwardly mobile, the next major source of stress usually occurs during their reintegration into the economy. (p. 568)

Another point raised in this paper and often overlooked when it is quoted, is that Brenner puts forward, in his penultimate paragraph, the idea that 'these instabilities in economic growth also account for the socio-economic differentials in mortality', and 'the mechanism by which unemployment and rapid economic growth act to slow the secular trend of mortality-rate decline is through a widening of the socio-economic differentials in mortality.' This was to provide a link at a later stage between the unemployment and health debate, and the debate on health inequalities. Very little of this complexity found its way into the public debate, either in media accounts of 'Death on the dole', or in parliamentary questions, although, in hindsight, many participants regarded the unemployment and health debate as 'just part of the debate on health inequalities'.[3]

The issue community develops

In other pieces of backstage activity, pressure-group participation in the issue community continued to take shape. By January of 1980, senior staff of the National Council for Voluntary Organisations (NCVO) had drawn up a proposal for a 'pilot study', to replicate Harvey Brenner's research in Britain. It was envisaged that the National Council for Social Service would employ two or three people to collate the necessary statistics, which would then be sent to Baltimore for analysis by Brenner's computer model.[4] It also proposed that a steering committee be set up, including representatives from NCSS and 'selected UK institutions'. A budget of £26,000 was estimated.

One participant in the events at this time explained the ability of Brenner's ideas to interest in the following way:

> NCVO was not very influential before ... [A new Director] came in as a young bright whizz kid and wanted to make his mark ... [Projects Department of the NCVO] was the department in which major growth was prized, because they could get small bits of money from the government to fund small pieces of work. Unemployment and health was one of the bright ideas ... It was a new idea, and they wanted to expand the Projects Division, it was seen as a way of getting money into the organisation.

In several accounts, therefore, the notion of 'having a bright idea and fighting for it' is used by participants from such diverse backgrounds as the media and the voluntary sector. This type of motivation for taking up the issue of the effect of unemployment on health was not greatly affected by the political colour of the party in power.

Also in early 1980, a new organisation was formed which was to have some influence upon the course of the debate. Jennie Popay, previously a staff member at USHP, had by now taken up a post at the Study Commission on the Family. She and a friend from student days who worked at the NCVO shared a long-standing interest in unemployment, first developed by their experiences studying social administration at Essex University. At the beginning of 1980 they began to promote the idea of a Social Costs of Unemployment Forum, with the support of the NCVO, whose purpose would be 'to collect and disseminate information to ... the increasing number of organisations and individuals at national and local levels [who] were acutely aware of the potential impact of unemployment but were unsure as to how to tackle the problem'.

Beginning with eight members, SCUF grew swiftly. By April it had thirty, including several members of the Radical Statistics Health Group, and community physicians of 'Manifesto' tendencies, and was beginning to be inundated with requests for information and speakers.

In the spring of 1980, Brenner renewed his contact with Liverpool by returning to address an EEC conference on 'urban social problems'. This time the invitation came from Alex Scott-Samuel who 'was anxious to expose the delegates to more than the comfortable lounge of a cushy hotel,' as he told journalist Steve Connor of *General Practitioner* (7 March 1980, p. 37) In June, the *Liverpool Daily Post* produced an exemplary piece of medical journalism on Brenner's work. It began with the 'human interest' angle, a tragic account of an individual's suicide, headlined 'Death of a good and willing worker'. Beneath was a series of clearly presented graphs adapted from *The Reckoning*. Granada, wrote David Utting, had brought Dr Brenner to Merseyside to see the human reality behind the statistics. Utting reported that Brenner had both pledged his 'active backing' to the NCVO proposal and expressed interest in Scott-Samuel's plan for an 'intensive study in a small area badly affected by unemployment.'

This latter point will have been a reference to the founding of another small group which was to be more persistent in its influence on the progress of the debate. This was the Unemployment and Health Study Group (UHSG), based in the recession-stricken North-West of England. They held their inaugural meeting, organised by Scott-Samuel, on 19 June. At their second meeting in September 1980, an MSc student in health economics from York University, Pat Kennan, spoke to the UHSG about the results of one of the DHSS-sponsored research projects which had been mentioned in parliamentary answers. This was her own Masters project, an attempt to replicate Brenner's econometric analysis on British statistics, supervised by an econometrician at Queen Mary College, London, Hugh Gravelle. This was eventually to form the basis of a paper which, a year later, spearheaded the scientific and official response to Brenner's claims.

The period 1977 to 1979 therefore saw 'the health of the unemployed' become established as a social problem worthy of attention from politicians, pressure groups, civil servants and the

media. There was little that could be called scientific activity
around the question during this time, however. Fagin and Little's
monograph and Brenner's paper provided the only original research relevant to the British situation. Draper *et al.*'s *Lancet* paper
was essentially a review and commentary. The low level of 'academic' activity around the issue which continued during 1980
cannot therefore be regarded as a result of the policies of the new
administration. One reason may be that 1980 was the year in
which the 'Black Report' on health inequalities between social
classes appeared, and attracted the attentions and energies of the
groups involved in health policy debate, although no explicit
connection was made between the two issues at this stage. A
considerable number of research proposals were also drawn up
during this period, none of which ever materialised into published work with impact on the debate.

A pilot study

In July 1980 the debate reappeared in the Commons when Labour
MP Dennis Skinner asked Patrick Jenkin, Secretary of State for
Social Services:

> if he will establish an urgent inquiry into the link between
> unemployment and heart diseases, mental stress, suicides
> and other health problems with particular reference to those
> areas in the country where unemployment ... is of a very
> high and long lasting nature.

In reply Jenkin assured Skinner that his department:

> is already involved in studies of health and the unemployed,
> including questions of their interrelation. We are also co-
> operating with outside researchers on a study of long-term
> unemployment and mortality ... We are aware of the re-
> search being done by Professor Brenner ... There is as yet no
> published work which establishes with any certainty a
> causative link between unemployment and ill health.
> (*Hansard* 20 July 1980, cols. 1276–7)

The 'outside research' referred to here was that being carried out
at Queen Mary College, London.

Another contribution to the debate was also in the process of
being produced at this time within the DHSS (and was referred to
in answer to another parliamentary question on unemployment
and health, by Renee Short on 1 August 1980). There was a
longitudinal study of unemployed men being conducted in the

department. This was the DHSS Cohort Study, from which Fagin
and Little had borrowed their sub-sample. This study was initiated in 1977, designed largely by Jon Stern, an economic adviser
in the Department, to allow econometric techniques to be used to
estimate the effects of unemployment benefits on the duration
and frequency of unemployment spells, as well as to measure the
'replacement ratio' of benefits to wages. In the third and final
interviewing 'sweep', some questions on health were 'tacked on',
with some misgivings as to their usefulness. The health questions
were intended to discover whether those men who had remained
unemployed for the full duration of the study had experienced
worse health than those who found work again. The results were
written up in a paper published in the *Employment Gazette* by two
economic advisers at the DHSS, Sue Ramsden and Clive Smee,
who reported that there was no significantly greater deterioration
in health among the men who found no new jobs.

However, neither of these new studies had reported by December of 1980, when Len Fagin and Martin Little submitted their
findings to the DHSS, the sponsors of their study. It seemed to
them a somewhat alarming experience, as they remembered it;
'we met a sort of committee in a very large room with one of those
huge round tables, like a NATO meeting, with a huge space
between 'us' and 'them' on the other side.' 'They' were 'about
twenty DHSS dignitaries' who 'used a lot of words like pilot,
descriptive, sampling methodological points.'

Fagin observed that in the public debate which followed,
'George Young and Gerard Vaughan ... used those exact comments, the very words that were used that day.' This insight into
the strategic dimension of official 'forms of words' was later
elaborated by a senior government research manager who considered it to be of the essence of the relationship between researcher
and political administrator. In answer to a question about how
researchers *inside* government maintained the boundary between
'fact' and 'opinion', she remarked that it was:

> a very fine line which was maintained in practice, by *lan-*
> *guage*. We draw the line by the use of very careful, heavy,
> official prose, an attempt to make things as factual and flat
> as possible ... [These forms of words] carry a lot of tacit
> meaning. Once they have been agreed, for example for use
> in an answer to a Parliamentary Question, they tend to be
> used over and over again.

The emphasis on the 'descriptive' nature of Fagin and Little's study had in fact been negotiated explicitly, in early 1979, between the researchers and the Central Statistical Office, whose Survey Control Unit has to give recognition to any survey carried out by government departments. There was a conflict between two aims shared by the researchers and the Control Unit. On the one hand, people responsible for the main Cohort Study (CS) did not want too many families to be interviewed by Fagin and Little (who no doubt had their own constraints of time and energy as well), in case this influenced the responses to the next sweep of the whole sample. On the other hand, the Control Unit had to urge the researchers to interview sufficient numbers of families to allow statistically meaningful comparisons to be made between, for example, those unemployed men whose wives were employed and those whose wives had no paid job. It was in response to this dilemma that Fagin himself had emphasised the 'descriptive' and 'pilot' aspects of his study.

The procedure for interviewing the twenty-two families reflected Fagin and Little's basic hypothesis, that families might be differentiated into 'good' and 'poor copers', those who had overcome previous life events (crises) with differing amounts of success. By adopting as one of its topics processes such as 'coping', the study design laid emphasis on individual rather than 'political' issues. Such an approach was congruent with the clinical approach adopted by the researchers, and seems unlikely to have led the civil servants who carried out the main project to anticipate that their report would produce political controversy. It is possible that in the absence of *The Reckoning* the reaction to the report might have been different.

There is more or less total disagreement between the researchers and the officials over what happened next to Fagin and Little's report. Fagin himself typed the report, so that 200 photocopies would be available for public consumption. These were duly issued by the DHSS – at least one research team wrote off for a copy to the DHSS headquarters at Elephant and Castle, and received one without delay. But Fagin felt that some attempt had been made to minimise the impact of the report. If this is true, it was a failed attempt. There is no example in the unemployment and health debate of a (real or suspected) attempt at 'government suppression of information' which failed to promote greater media interest than would have been aroused in its absence. Pressure groups (and, increasingly, academics) know this, so that there is some temptation to imply a 'cover-up' in order to gain the attention of journalists.

Officials who spoke frankly about departmental activity in the unemployment and health debate were insistent that there was no attempt to limit the availability of the report. On 9 June 1981, Sir George Young made a statement in the House of Commons in reply to several questions from Labour MPS about Fagin and Little's work. The researchers were not happy with the statement. Fagin took Young to task for failing sufficiently to emphasise that although the health of two men had admittedly improved after they became unemployed, a deterioration in health was found in more families. At the same time, he asked that the DHSS lower the price of the report (£6) and make more copies available. Young gave a long and considered reply, stressing that in his statement he had admitted that 'it seemed reasonable to assume that there is some association between unemployment and health' and that he had been 'simply pointing out the difficulty of drawing clear conclusions about cause and effect' from a small study.

Shortly afterwards, Fagin also had to reproach the editor of the *News of the World* for what he felt had been a 'sensationalised' report of the study's findings, published on 16 August. The argument died down during the summer parliamentary recess, but re-emerged in October when a group of Labour MPs, organised by the Junior Opposition Spokesman on health, asked a battery of oral questions on unemployment and health (*Hansard*, 20 October 1981, cols. 154–6). Dr Gerard Vaughan, then Minister for Health, had the task of replying. Like Young's, Vaughan's replies angered Fagin, who felt that the Minister had 'misguided Parliament ... for what I can only conceive are political purposes'. Even so, it was not the accuracy of Vaughan's statement that Fagin quarrelled with, but rather its emphasis. Rather than taking the acknowledged preliminary nature of the research as an indication that more and bigger studies were needed, the fact that it had been 'only a pilot' was being used to minimise the importance of the findings. In his reply to Fagin, Vaughan spoke of the research at Queen Mary College (Gravelle's work with Pat Kennan) and the CS as responses to the need for more knowledge, and made rather vague references to 'fresh work designed to clarify the nature and significance of any unemployment-health links ... with the benefit of expert advice from independent sources'.

This correspondence between Fagin and Vaughan was placed in the House of Commons Library in mid-November, and, after another small flurry of letters between Fagin, the Labour MPs who asked the original questions, and Vaughan, the matter rested there. By this time, also, major developments had taken place in the academic debate, which will be discussed below.

Fagin himself, three years later, felt that the major impact of his and Little's work had been on other professional groups, rather than on policy-makers. Another effect he felt was that, by 1984, the media tended far less to treat the unemployed as 'scroungers' and more to admit that unemployment could not be the fault of individuals. This had also been part of the purpose of the CS as a whole, to investigate the question of the 'replacement ratio' in order to see whether a large proportion of the unemployed were indeed 'better off on the dole', as some headlines in the late 1970s had described them (Moylan *et al*, 1984). In the longer term, therefore, the impact of the smaller study (as perceived by Fagin) and the larger one of which it was a part were, in this sense at least, consistent and in the desired direction.

During 1979 and 1980, therefore, links began to be forged which were to persist and to influence not only the unemployment and health controversy, but the future of the 'Radical' ginger group in community medicine, the activity of research teams in the field of population statistics, public health and epidemiology, and Labour party health policy. In tracing out the history of these links, we will begin to see the extent to which the arguments presented in the debate were constructed in a context of wider strategies pursued by the complex of groups involved. 'Unemployment and health' was a vehicle for diverse groups' and individuals' projects, as well as a topic in its own right. The activity of the USHP in informing interested MPs, Granada Television in making *The Reckoning* and Brenner and Fagin and Little in publishing the results of their research appeared to have uncovered a social problem. The problem was interpreted not only by the media but also by academics as the damaging effect of the experience of unemployment on the physical and/or mental health of the unemployed. As we have seen, Brenner's paper said something rather more complex, but this model of the relationship between health and economy did not receive any further attention for many years. The pressure groups which had become involved were small and new. However, two more groups now became involved which was to add considerably to the impetus of Brenner's ideas.

Notes

1. Mr Golding will have had the benefit of professional advice from a research group located within the Department of Employment which was at this time very highly respected academically.
2. To take three members of either the 'Rethinking Community Medicine' author group and/or the group around Radical Community Medicine, John Dennis of USHP was active within the Labour Party as an adviser on health and related issues, Jennie Popay, who worked at USHP during the making of *The Reckoning* and Alex Scott-Samuel became members of a 'Front Bench Advisory Group' on health, convened by Michael Meacher, the Shadow Secretary of State for Health and Social Security, in the summer of 1984. Later, they both became members of the official health sub-committee of the Labour Party National Executive which drew up the health proposals for the 1987 election.
3. An attempt to place these considerations more centrally in the early debate failed, as reported in Chapter 3 below.
4. The proposal not to analyse the data in Britain is, of course, an indication of the extent to which Brenner's 'model' had become a 'black box', to British researchers.

3

THE CELTIC 'FRINGE'

The Cardiff conference

In 1981, two pressure groups adopted the unemployment and health issue, without whose promotion it is doubtful whether the work of Brenner would have continued to have quite the same amount of impact. These were the Welsh and Scottish National Parties which, for various reasons (Drucker and Brown 1980, Clarke and Drucker 1978) were in a relatively active phase of their own development at this time. The idea that unemployment could harm health was particularly striking to them because of the way in which unemployment is regionally distributed in Britain.

Only one of these conferences had an impact on the subsequent development of the academic debate. This was sponsored by the Welsh National Party and took place on 10 April 1981 in Cardiff. Speakers included a mixture of political medical and social-science 'names'. Brenner duly put in a well-publicised appearance. The conference was attended by a wide range of experts from all over Britain, as well as local activists. Speakers included leading academic figures such as Prof George Brown, co-author of *Social Origins of Depression* and the leading British authority on life event research, and prominent members of the local medical community, as well as a consultant psychiatrist associated with the Welsh National Party, and a research officer for the Wales TUC. In the words of its organiser Dr Stephen Farrow, a Senior Lecturer in Community Medicine at the Welsh National School, his objective for the conference was 'to put Social Medicine back on the agenda of my own Department.' The unanticipated furore which it caused, including an American camera team, was not, for that reason, unwelcome although it may not have been strictly intended.

Although the Cardiff conference was planned as a claims-making exercise, aimed at influencing both the theory and practice of community medicine, and wider public opinion on government policy, the most lasting result of what took place was a contribution to the moral and technical fragmentation of the issue. A *Lancet* editorial wrote of the conference (18 April 1981):

The causal chain – from economic depression through organic illness to premature death is instinctively believable ... [but] over the teacups there were serious criticisms of Brenner's findings: UK workers do not seem to be able to confirm his work, but this criticism is not yet, as the Americans would say, in the public domain.

One of the events that took place over the teacups was an encounter between a deputy editor of *The Lancet* and an economist whose career had included spells working as a government adviser (on the CS amongst other projects). As he remembered:

I went down there [to Cardiff] and watched the NBC cameras and all the carry-on. [two colleagues] were there too. We sat ourselves in the first two or three rows. Brenner said the Cohort Study results missed the point as most of the effects of unemployment were not on the unemployed themselves but on the health of the non-unemployed. Well, this I could not understand ... It was just his way of dismissing the Cohort Study results. After tea, a man came up to me and said he liked my question ... he turned out to be the deputy editor of *The Lancet*. I asked if he would welcome a paper on this.

The suggestion by the editor of *The Lancet* that a high-status medical journal might 'welcome' papers by economists on unemployment and health was an important step in the shaping of the next stage of the 'technical' debate.

The Scottish National Party conference

During 1979–81, because of USHP's funding problems, Peter Draper was having fairly intensive discussions with the members of the Unit's Steering Committee, and other senior advisers. This group included several prominent figures in the Scottish health policy field: Sir John Brotherston, ex-Chief Medical Officer for Scotland and Emeritus Professor of Community Medicine at Edinburgh University, Dr John Loraine, an eminent endocrinologist in semi-retirement who headed Edinburgh's Centre for Human Ecology, Dr David Player, Director of the Scottish Health Education Group since 1975, and Mr T. Drummond Hunter, Secretary of the Scottish Health Services Planning Group. Some of these people also had sympathies with the ideals of

Scottish nationalism, more specifically with the notion that there
was something special about the Scottish approach to community
medicine, as reflected in the Gilloran Report (Joint Working Party
1973). By early 1981 (before Cardiff), there had been links established between Peter Draper, David Player, Sir John, a senior
medical officer in the Scottish Home and Health Department, and
Iain More, a full-time worker for the Scottish National Party.

The connection between USHP thinking and that of a certain
group of Scottish health planners and policy advisers was centred
around a set of ideas less directly related to devolution, perhaps
exemplified by Drummond Hunter's 1976 paper on The Reorganised Health Service in Clarke and Drucker's book *Our Changing
Scotland*:

> In Scotland [he wrote] a more imaginative stance [on the
> 1974 health service reorganisation], which may have reflected
> oft-repeated views of the CMO, Sir John Brotherston, was
> adopted ... reorganisation in Scotland was not simply an
> attempt on the part of government to regain control of a
> runaway health service. (p. 31) Health ... has less to do with
> services than with life-chances and life-styles. (p. 35)

It was the uniqueness of the USHP that it briefly attempted to
combine all these issues in its work. The ideas came together into
the Glasgow conference scheme because of largely informal links
between some of the initiators, a fact perhaps reflected in the
constant good-natured references to 'a Mafia'.

For the senior medical officer, it had been his political ideas
and contacts which lay behind his interest in the issue:

> We [self, player and Brotherston] are a sort of Mafia. The
> SNP [had] taken a political and psychological knock [by the
> combined effects of the failure of the devolution vote in 1979
> and the return of a right wing government] ... we were
> using unemployment and health as a political issue. In fact, I
> now think this was wrong. It should have been used not as a
> party issue, but as an evil in itself.

Iain More explained:

> There were 3 people in the SHHD who had done some sort
> of studies on unemployment and health and [one of them] is
> on the policy committee of the SNP. We thought that a
> quality conference with a minimum of party politics would
> be a good thing, at least that was my first idea. We [SNP]
> would then get the credit for it ... Brenner appeared to be

the most outstanding person in the field. So I wrote to him. He was interested. He said he'd be across in the UK for that conference in Cardiff ... We [SNP] try to do one thing like this every year ... You need to build up credibility in the eyes of opinion makers. Short term things are most important to political groups like the SNP ... You get your mileage out of something like this and then lose interest.

More expressed some conflict between his own 'intellectual fascination' with the question and commitment to finding short-term problems to which SNP policies could be offered as plausible answers, one of the organisational exigencies of his professional role. According to one colleague David Player's own personal history meant that 'he was conscious of Scotland's health problems ... He was generally concerned. He is a close friend of Peter Draper's and Gerry Morris's ... They are a bit of a Glasgow Mafia really.' So there appear to have been institutional (through the Steering Committee of USHP), philosophical, political (through the SNP and wider group of nationalist sympathisers), and informal links between the leading figures behind the Glasgow conference (they were 'golfing buddies' according to one participant). As well as being seen as a 'good political issue', unemployment and health articulated several concerns common to community medicine, health education, health economics and NHS planning, and thereby 'enrolled' actors from all these areas into a new, fragile network. This was the source of the impact of Brenner's ideas in these professional circles.

However, several participants in the organisation of the Glasgow conference later expressed a view that using Brenner's work too uncritically and too 'politically' had perhaps been a mistake. The two academics invited to the conference in order to debate directly with Brenner were Steve Engelman, a senior lecturer in health economics at Edinburgh Medical School's department of community medicine, and Mike Porter, the medical school's sociology lecturer, also an economist by training. Like Porter and the USHP staff, Engelman had been finding Brenner's work useful in teaching, since the late 1970s. Engelman's memory was that Brenner's work was not, at this time, thought to be particularly controversial, but he had thought it 'interesting', and the sort of thing medical students ought to know about. From the technical point of view, like other economists, Engelman realised Brenner's work was 'econometrically unsatisfactory' but that it had 'potential shock-horror value'. As he put it, 'usually, econometric work has problems, but other people take it up and work on it and either it improves or it gets forgotten.'

In the short term, the outcome of the Glasgow conference satisfied at least some of the organisers. Like the USHP, the SNP succeeded in presenting Brenner's work as subsidised information – the press and TV took the bait. However, as a non-party, academic conference aimed at serious consideration of evidence on a public health issue, the outcome was less favourable. One academic described Brenner's speech as a 'disaster', and another gave a scathing account:

> It was terrible to be preached at like that for so long … it was like an evangelical meeting, no one had a chance to talk back. Oh yes, they gave Harvey Brenner a chance to talk back and we got more figures and charts and he unfolded all this other data. He tried to blind people with figures any time anyone tried to make a point … It wasn't fair.

Instead of being seen as technical virtuosity, Brenner's complex methods and large volume of data are now referred to as 'preaching' and 'blinding' people with data. Iain More admitted to having faced some criticism for his use of Brenner as centre piece: 'it was suggested to me that by using Brenner we could destroy the issue … The argument was that people interested in the politics were not really interested in serious research'.

At the end of the conference, Richard Smith, an assistant editor at the *British Medical Journal (BMJ)* and a graduate of Edinburgh University's medical school, highlighted the non-academic agenda of the conference for his readers by reminding them that Sir John Brotherston had called for 'a Scottish forum where issues like this one that are especially important for Scotland could be debated.' As in Cardiff, the 'scientific' issue had been perhaps more important as a vehicle for Nationalist policies. Accordingly, academic participants in the conference were not optimistic about the possibilities for 'further research', despite the frequent mentions of research in answers to Parliamentary Questions at this time. Steve Engelman and a colleague at Glasgow University, John Forbes, put in a proposal subsequently to the Scottish Health Services Research Committee,[1] although they were aware that this topic was, as Engelman put it 'not health *services* research but I thought it was of considerable public interest.' The £120–130,000 they had asked for was, Engelman realised, a lot of money, but the only appropriate method was an expensive longitudinal design 'if you're really going to throw any light on the matter'. Despite having lowered their original financial estimate, their application was not successful (but for an account of the fate of Forbes and Engelman's proposal from within Whitehall, see Chapter 4).

John Forbes saw the future for research in the area quite clearly:

> We tried [himself and Engelman] to get a proposal together [in 1982]. The Scottish Office said they didn't have the money, they sent it to the Dept of Employment, the DHSS, all around the place. It was just after the [1983] General Election that they wrote back saying it had been given low priority ... Now, I feel it is curious the way they turned it down. They might have jacked it on methodological grounds or said it was not do-able. One way you might get them to support your research might be to say you believed there were econometric problems with any existing piece of work which seemed to show an effect. This can always be done: 'Dear Minister, We think there are problems with Brenner ...' But as soon as you get a rejection like this one, you lose interest. It is a big investment that has gone to nothing.

These comments illustrate the process by which researchers make use of the prominence given to a topic by policy debates to 'inter-' est' funding bodies and generate support for future research. It shows how researchers, activists and professionals puzzle over which alliances are the best ones to seek, which groups need to be 'interested' and what is the best way of accomplishing that aim. The difficulty of choosing the best strategy is further illustrated in the fate of the next Scottish conference on unemployment and health.

The Stirling 'consultation'

The Edinburgh Medical Group Consultation 'Work, health and high unemployment', which took place on 1–3 June 1982, had been in planning stage almost since the beginning of the Glasgow planning process. Unlike Glasgow, which had been put together by Iain More and a member of staff at the Scottish Health Education Group (SHEG), Stirling had a Steering Group, which held its first meeting on 23 April 1981. The purpose of the Stirling 'consultation' as it was termed, was 'to be complementary to Glasgow

rather than competing.' It was seen as a more overtly 'political'
event, in that political subjects would be explicitly raised, instead
of being implied by the factual claims presented as 'research'.
And yet, in its organisation it was far *less* 'political' – no particular
party or pressure group was involved – Iain More was invited to
give advice only. A colleague of Player's at SHEG related 'Stirling
was an attempt to provide a responsibe medical basis for the
unemployment and health debate ... Dr Player saw that there was
another dimension the debate, an economic and political as well
as an epidemiological argument'.

Although David Player and others regarded Stirling as 'less
political' than Glasgow, the Scottish Office were not convinced. In
May 1982, a letter arrived at SHEG from Scottish Office headquarters at St Andrews House which criticised Player for becoming
involved in the Stirling conference. The letter's author (a civil
servant, not a politician) wrote:

> I know you will not take it amiss if I offer my strong per-
> sonal view that it is stretching the Group's role well beyond
> the limits that the Management Committee [of SHEG] are
> likely to endorse ... What is the health education point? If
> unemployment is bad for health, are health educators to
> argue for higher levels of employment than the combined
> wisdom of economists, industrialists, and politicians would
> otherwise achieve? If it should transpire that unemploy-
> ment is sometimes good for health, is SHEG to be in the
> business of pressing for Government health warnings on
> appropriate pay packets?

The letter's author in fact puts his finger squarely on the point that
Peter Draper and his USHP co-workers, the 'Re-Thinking Community Medicine' team, the group around *Radical Community
Medicine* and the UHSG had been trying to make since 1979 by
using Brenner's work on health and the economy. That is, the
claim that a true 'community medicine' should be involved in
wider issues of policy and politics.

There was disagreement, however, among the conference's
organising group, over what sort of alliance between 'medicine',
'science' and 'social policy' should be pursued. Some organisers
and speakers felt that the major theme of the conference should be
'inequality' and that the links should be drawn more explicitly
than in Glasgow between general issues (both 'scientific' and
'political') of inequality and the question of the health of the

unemployed. One speaker, Chris Pond (director of the Low Pay Unit) later explained:

> there is a close link between unemployment and low pay. I am critical of some of the work on unemployment and health as it sees unemployment as something discrete ... Really there is a spectrum from the casual worker to the well-paid, permanently employed person with a whole range in between. So the [Low Pay] Unit can't afford to ignore unemployment.

This theme was also reflected in other contributions to the consultation. One speaker, Prof Bernard Crick, had previously written, 'Certainly, if there was no difference in the death rate between social classes, we would know that we no longer had social classes' (Crick 1982, p. 225). He told the Stirling audience:

> The Black Report has established that ill-health is bad enough for the lowest social classes compared to the higher classes even when in jobs, but unemployment is associated with poverty not merely absolutely but also relatively. There may be no direct evidence that unemployment creates ill health, but the evidence is overwhelming that poverty creates ill-health. (*Contact* no. 76, 1983:3 p. 12)

In David Player's contribution, he concluded

> those of us in the NHS should try to do something about social class inequalities in health along the lines recommended by the Black Report ... If social class inequalities in health could be tackled many unemployed people would benefit. (*Contact* no, 76, 1983:3 p. 8).

This might seem to portray the beginnings of a promising alliance between political scientists, 'neo-Keynesian' economists (as Pond described himself) and a segment of the medical profession represented by Player. However, what the extracts from conference papers published in *Contact* (the journal of the Scottish Pastoral Association and Clinical Theology Association) reflect is the outcome of a conflict within the steering group over the orientation of the conference.

In an informal discussion on 28 September of 1981, during the planning process for the Consultation, one senior academic had expressed concern at the lack of connection between those studying health and those studying the effects of recession on living standards and the labour market. Minutes of this meeting note that he had instanced the separation of studies on unemployment, redundancy, and chronic poverty, also the split in academic and government departments between the various interests of health, economics, sociology and social administration. These concerns come near to echoing (almost certainly unintentionally) Brenner's theme that unemployment strikes hardest at those already most vulnerable, and exerts its effects on health by increasing inequalities in living standards. Although this theme was prominent in many of the papers, both those reported in *Contact* and those which were not, it was not reflected in the (rather scant) public reporting of the consultation. Nor was it remembered by many of the participants interviewed later. The question of social inequality did not re-appear with any prominence in the unemployment and health debate until some three years later.

Some on the organising committee interpreted the references to the importance of poverty and inequality as an attempt by the 'poverty lobby' to over-influence the agenda of the consultation. This, it was felt, might militate against unemployment and health being seen as a vehicle for enrolling 'responsible medical' opinion. As one participant saw it:

> The social consequences of unemployment are hard to measure, but medical data is different, lay people trust it more, it has more legitimacy ... thought it was very important to use doctors and epidemiological information – it would be more effective if we had doctors ... than the same old, tired battery of activists ... wanted a new medical dimension ... people who were uncontaminated by identification with a particular political line [such as] the left wing crowd from the Study Commission on the Family and the Low Pay Unit.

Only much later was it to be suggested that consideration of wider questions concerning social inequality might be a way out of the academic impasse into which the debate now descended (for an interpretation of the research using this approach see Bartley 1988, 1991). For the time being, any association between those promoting the involvement of the medical profession in the social problem of the health of the unemployed and those who had for long been analysing and commenting upon inequalities in, for example, income, working conditions and security of work was seen as undesirable by the former group.

It was the simple link between unemployment and mortality which had both 'interested' the medical profession and gained media coverage. By diverging from this theme the organisers of the Stirling conference, despite the generally acknowledged quality of the speakers and their contributions, took the risk of reducing the power of the issue to help social scientists enrol doctors. By hazarding the support of such a powerful group, a real risk was posed to the potential impact the conference might have on the public debate and thereby on policy-makers' views of 'what research was needed' at that stage.

Note

1. A body whose *raison d'être* was similar to that of the CSRC and MRC Health Services Research Panel discussed in Part 2.

4

EVIDENCE AND CIRCUMSTANCES

The official response to Brenner

Although the Cardiff and Glasgow conferences in 1981 may be regarded as the point at which Brenner's ideas reached their maximum impact in Britain, the Glasgow conference was also the first public confrontation between Brenner and his British critics. The evening before the Glasgow conference, a small invitation-only seminar was held at the University in which Brenner debated directly with two of his critics: Stern and Gravelle. They had been horrified to hear, in the taxi from Glasgow station, a radio item stating that 'An American academic produces new research showing that unemployment will kill 70,000 in Scotland this year'. There was an impression among those less technically minded members of the small audience that Brenner had not successfully defended his work. The attack by Gravelle and Stern may be regarded as the opening shots in the second phase of the debate: the 'official response'.

This response had been developing for some time, probably since the screening of Granada's *The Reckoning* programme in early 1979. In November of 1980 Brenner came to Britain for a tour which included testimony to the House of Lords Select Committee on Unemployment. During this time the *Guardian*'s economic correspondent Frances Cairncross interviewed him, and the resulting article was written in a sceptical vein. Cairncross was obviously well aware of the work in progress at Queen Mary College, although this was not to be published for almost another year. She also quotes research from the Policy Studies Institute showing that 90 per cent of all people who became unemployed in the year 1979 had left the register within six months. She wrote in the *Guardian* of 7 November 1980:

> Those who remained out of work for long periods could almost be predicted in advance: they tended to be older workers, unskilled, with poor mental or physical health.

> They are precisely the people who, for a whole host of other
> reasons, would tend to have exceptionally high sickness and
> mortality rates.

This concentration upon the question of 'who, in terms of health,
are the unemployed?', was referred to by one DHSS adviser as
'the *ceteris paribus* argument'. It was completely implausible, he
felt, that a reduction in the unemployment rate could lower the
national mortality rate. And yet this is what Brenner's work
seemed to be implying. Was it not more likely that other things
made the unemployed untypical such that, if all other things were
equal, if they were not unemployed, they would still have characteristics which might tend to cause ill-health? This argument was
to figure prominently in the future progress of the debate. Yet set
in temporal context it can be seen that Brenner's work in itself did
not necessarily justify such an emphasis. In the autumn of 1980,
no-one had produced an academic paper claiming to demonstrate
that individual unemployed persons were adversely affected in
health (this was to come in Fagin and Little's monograph). As an
economist herself, it may be that Cairncross had access to information on how certain of her colleagues intended to steer the
debate, and her relatively small article, placed in an inconspicu-
ous position in the newspaper, marks an important turning point.

A young economist working at USHP during this time,
Howard Cox, remembered that:

> When [Brenner] made that return visit, his work was al-
> ready coming under fire. The main criticism seemed to be
> that he looked at an atypical time period. I told him I didn't
> think it would wear ... was conscious of a critical attitude
> the first time I mentioned Brenner's name in a group of
> economists.

Whereas 1981 may perhaps be regarded as the high point of the
public debate, political controversy and government response
and of Brenner's influence, it was also the period in which credibility in Brenner's work was steadily undermined. On 3 April
1981 the DHSS put out an official press release of a speech to be
delivered by Sir George Young, then Undersecretary of State for
Health, to the Conference of Northern Region Community Health
Councils. It may have been knowledge of the forthcoming Cardiff
conference which precipitated the content of Young's speech, and
the drawing of attention to such a relatively minor event. The
speech was the first example of a careful information subsidy on

'the health of the unemployed' produced by the Department of
Health under a Conservative administration. It was headed:

> *Possible link between unemployment and ill-health*
> *deeply concerns ministers*

and went on:

> Sir George said that two relevant research projects were
> commissioned by the Department some time ago and a third
> had been commissioned more recently. 'I understand they
> [the results] are likely to suggest that there is little or no
> causal relationship between unemployment and health ...
> where the duration of the unemployment is less than one
> year ... The median period of unemployment for the indi-
> vidual who goes on to the register is still comparatively
> short, about three months. So far as possible, we should be
> aiming our help at the minority who reach ... the third stage,
> when depression sets in: these are often the people who are
> at a disadvantage already, perhaps for health reasons, or
> perhaps because they are old, or unskilled.

By 7 July 1981 (provoked by a somewhat heated exchange in
the House of Commons over the Fagin Report, as described in
chapter 2), the backstage progress of Brenner's collaboration with
his new found British enthusiasts was appearing in the public
forum once again. Nigel Duncan wrote in Pulse (7 July 1981):

> For a long time the field has been left largely to an American
> research scientist, Prof Harvey Brenner of Johns Hopkins
> University ... But there have been a number of criticisms of
> his work ... The DHSS is now sponsoring its own research at
> Queen Mary College to see if it can repeat Brenner's findings
> ... But the findings will only show associations between
> unemployment and death rates. They cannot show causal-
> ity, the effect of unemployment on health, and it is this
> which many people believe is of far greater importance.

In the 'News' section of the same edition of the journal, Duncan
wrote of suspicions that the DHSS was deliberately trying to
muffle debate on the issue by limiting the availability of the Fagin
Report. On the 23 July, the *Guardian* and *New Society* referred to
the unemployment and health issue. *New Society* (23 July 1981)
commented: 'There hasn't been a lot of critical evaluation of
[Brenner's] findings. Some people have been concerned ... that,
should Brenner's work not be substantiated, politicians who

wished to play down the effects of unemployment would have a field day.'

On 1 August 1981, *The Lancet* published a letter by Brenner which included figures for England, Wales and Scotland, referring to the major critique which the group of economists were developing, to the effect that the equations used to describe the 1936–76 relationship between economic and mortality figures failed to hold up when applied outside of this specific time period. Brenner promises work on 'trends in mortality for several major causes in England and Wales and Scotland during the period 1950 to 1978' which 'confirm the main conclusions of the earlier report on England and Wales ... for the post-war period in England, Wales and Scotland, unemployment rates, specified for age, sex and duration of unemployment are strongly associated with increased death rates' (for the eventual results of these studies see Brenner and Mooney 1982, 1983; Brenner 1983). Howard Cox wrote to Brenner that this analysis would 'make Gravelle *et al.*'s critique of your earlier paper redundant.'

The results of the the the inquiry into the effect of unemployment on health by the DHSS's own 'Cohort Study of the unemployed' were published in the *Employment Gazette* on 24 September 1981 (Ramsden and Smee 1981). The official press release sums up the paper:

> This is the first British study to examine this possible link using data from a national survey ... and accepts that an association [between unemployment and health] is not disputed. What is disputed is whether unemployment itself causes ill-health. Unhealthy people may well be more likely to lose their jobs and have difficulty finding a new one: the worse the sickness record, the less the chance of re-employment.

The paper advertised in this press release illustrated these claims with figures comparing the health of those members of the DHSS unemployed cohort who had found new jobs with that of those who had remained unemployed during the whole period of the study. The latter group's self-reported health did not appear to have been any more likely to deteriorate than the health of those re-employed.

On 26 September the results of the Queen Mary College study by Hugh Gravelle, Gillian Hutchinson and Jon Stern was published in *The Lancet*. Brenner's work, they argue:

is important because it suggests that the social costs of unemployment may be higher than has previously been
thought. Further [they claim, somewhat surprisingly] time
series analysis can provide a fairly precise estimate of how
much mortality rates would rise following a given increase
in unemployment. (Gravelle *et al.*, 1981)

The first section of the paper concentrates on firstly, the 1930s
studies and secondly, what Brenner had claimed in Cardiff on 10
April. It specifically disputes the point that 'high unemployment
is associated with declines in real income for the employed as well
as the unemployed.' This scholarly if brief review then tackles the
problem that cross-sectional studies tend to *support* the notion of a
correlation between measures of unemployment and mortality in
different geographical areas. However, the reader is reminded
that:

these studies typically find that a number of other variables
such as income, occupational structure, educational levels,
consumption patterns and housing are also associated with
mortality and that these variables are strongly correlated
with unemployment rates. If these other variables are included in the analysis, the reliability (in terms of standard
errors) of the estimates of the effect of unemployment will
be reduced ... on the other hand, if these other variables are
omitted, the estimates will be biased, in that some of the
effects of omitted variables on mortality will be wrongly
attributed to unemployment. (Gravelle *et al.* 1981)

The argument here is that the apparent association between *unemployment* and health is more likely to be due to the types of job,
housing, education and 'consumption' such as diet, smoking and
drinking characteristic of people who become (or remain) unemployed. What the economists were aware of long before other
disciplines was the 'segmentation' of the British Labour market
(commented on by for example Hakim 1982, who was the only
non-economist to point out the possible significance of this to the
debate on 'health'). In 1979 Stern had published a paper entitled
'Who bears the burden of unemployment?' which showed how
unevenly the risk of unemployment is distributed throughout the
workforce. A very high proportion of the total amount of 'days
unemployment' in any given period of time are in fact experienced by a relatively small number of people, either as single long
spells or as a pattern of intermittent work. Sinfield had previously

described this as 'in and out of work', and later the phrase 'chequered work history' was coined by a research team investigating the consequences of large scale redundancy in South Wales (Harris, Lee and Morris 1985; Lee 1985, Fevre 1987; Harris 1987). Research had also suggested that people at high risk of unemployment could be heavier smokers and drinkers than those at lower risk. It was the latter possibility, that higher rates of illness and mortality in 'the unemployed' could be a result of consumption patterns, which became part of the subsequent debate.

The tone is set here for all the subsequent attacks on Brenner's work. The rest of the paper is highly technical (as was Brenner's original paper), was barely understood even by medical statisticians, and must have been opaque to the majority of the medical readership of *The Lancet*. But communication of detailed technique was not the purpose of the paper, and is therefore not necessary for an understanding of the role played by the economists' arguments in the wider debate. The task they performed, despite the complexity of their papers throughout the debate, was not one of 'technical fragmentation' but rather of 'individualization' (in Manning's terms). In essence, they argued that people who were found to be unemployed were always 'different' to those employed (other things were *not* equal), and that this difference resided in the possible pre-existing ill health of the employed and in individual characteristics such as health-related behavior, intelligence, and other aspects of 'human capital'. Unemployment might be directly harmful to a few, but most of the ill health in this group would have been there anyway.

The argument did contain an element of 'technical' fragmentation, almost literally. This was the importance of the 'once for all' change in both mortality and unemployment rates which took place at the end of the Second World War. In statistical terms, these two sharp changes were so large as to determine the value of the equation linking mortality and unemployment over the whole time period 1936–76, so that if one attempts to apply the same model to time periods which exclude the post-war period, or which split the period 1936–76 in two, it fails. In political terms, this argument marks out the professional territory of the economists within the welfare complex. They were arguing, in effect, that the welfare state had brought about a decisive improvement in health, such that any analysis of the much smaller changes in the periods before and after 1945 was of little relevance. Gravelle,

Hutchinson and Stern conclude: 'his [Brenner's] evidence does not support the hypothesis that aggregate unemployment rates have a serious adverse effect on population mortality rates.' The authors caution: 'Our results ... do *not* mean that unemployment has no adverse health effects. Indeed it is plausible that such effects do exist – but there is as yet no evidence which can be used to estimate their magnitude, timing and form.'

The effect of these two papers on the public debate conducted by pressure groups was to damp it down very considerably. On 3 October 1981, the ever-alert *Pulse* journalist Nigel Duncan reported:

> A major new row has broken out over unemployment and ill-health and the government's role in the affair ... Both reports [Ramsden and Smee and GH&S] will be welcomed by ministers and will harden their controversial refusal to accept any link between ill-health and unemployment ... critics of the government [were] describing them as deliberate attempts to discredit the growing campaign which sees unemployment as a major threat to public health. [This] comes just five weeks before Brenner is due to produce a major new analysis on unemployment and health in Scotland ... DHSS officials hope that critical scrutiny of Brenner's work will inject an element of caution into the debate.

On 20 October a series of Parliamentary Questions were asked about Len Fagin and Martin Little's report (see Chapter 2) and other research into unemployment and health which the government was suspected of manipulating. Gerard Vaughan told Dale Campbell-Savours that the work of the research team at Queen Mary College 'calls into question the validity of the statistical model used by Professor Brenner since it fails to take account of the relevant factors such as improvement in diet and medical care which occurred during the period' (*Hansard* 20 October 1981 WA col (10)97).

Gravelle *et al.* had called Brenner's bluff in using his own complicated methods against him. They had, to some extent, broken open the technical 'black box' represented by the time-series analysis. Gravelle and his colleagues' rebuttal of Brenner and Ramsden and Smee's paper from the DHSS Cohort Study therefore opened the 'official response' to the use made by 'Manifesto' community medicine and pressure groups of Brenner's work. The failure of the DHSS to produce a more formal version of the Fagin report (and the fact that there only 200 were made available), and ministerial denial in the House of Commons that the report demonstrated any 'causal' effect were taken, by some participants, to be another indication of official opposition. Also, media interest was, at this time, beginning to shift from the effect of unemployment on health itself to the (sometimes thrillingly unseemly) conflicts between doctors and ministers, and the associated accusations of 'cover-up'.

New research: entering the loop

By the autumn of 1981, the unemployment and health debate could be seen as having entered a 'loop' of claim and counter-claim. Calls for more research had been loud in Parliament, even after the Gravelle and Ramsden papers, and as it happened there were three research teams in a position to provide a certain amount even without new funding. Their results now began to appear quite quickly. The three studies which proved of greatest importance to the debate all made their first contributions during 1982.

The first of these was from the British Regional Heart Study, a large prospective study of heart disease aetiology. This study had carried out interviews and clinical examinations on approximately 350 men between the ages of 40 and 59 in each of twenty-four British towns between mid-1978 and mid-1980. The questionnaire collected details of present state of health (so that the researchers knew not only what diseases, if any, each man was suffering from, but also whether he and his doctor knew about them), diet, exercise, smoking, drinking. In order to be available for use as a control variable, information on occupation and employment status had also been collected. The researchers had found that 31 per cent of the unemployed, as compared to 15 per cent of the employed men had bronchitis; 28 per cent of the unemployed versus 15 per cent of the employed had obstructive lung disease; and 26 per cent of the unemployed, in contrast to 9 per cent of the employed had chest pain indicative of ischaemic heart disease. It was then necessary to allow for the fact that so many of the BRHS men without jobs were unemployed *because* of their ill health. Doing this changed the picture considerably. The 'not ill unemployed' were far less likely than the 'ill unemployed' to be suffering from symptoms suggestive of heart and lung disease. There was still some difference between the employed and the unemployed, though this was further decreased when statistical adjustment was made for social class, town of residence and smoking. However, even then, men unemployed for reasons other than ill health were still significantly more likely than the employed to have chest pain indicative of heart disease. The paper also questioned its own technique of adjusting for social class. Why was this done? Because every epidemiologist knows that mortality is related to class. However, it is possible that one reason for this is that the uneven class distribution of unemployment (pointed out by Sinfield and also by Stern in earlier work) may be one reason for the higher mortality in less advantaged classes. In this case there was a risk of controlling out the effect they were looking for.

A version of the paper was presented at the BSA Medical Sociology Conference in September 1981 where it caused little comment. In late March 1982 it was submitted it to *The Lancet* (Cook *et al.* 1982). It was accepted without major alteration, and published on 6 June. Somewhat to the authors' surprise (and disappointment), the appearance of the paper caused very little media comment, a few column inches on an inside page of the *Guardian*.

The second piece of research to enter the public domain (on 9 June) was a monograph presenting first results of an official study carried out as part of the work done by the Office of Population Censuses and Surveys, the OPCS Longitudinal Study. This study ('the LS') had linked 1971 Census information (including employment status) on 1 per cent of the population of England and Wales to births and deaths in the years 1971 to 1976. This was a very large study (the sample size was half a million individuals) and the first attempt in Britain[1] to link information on individuals gathered at a census to future life events. It reported that the results showed a death rate from accidents and violent causes, including suicide, amongst the unemployed well over twice as high as that for men in work, and a death rate from cancer half again as high as that for the employed[2] (Fox and Goldblatt 1982). It did not provoke any great media response: an article on page 2 of *The Times* headed 'Unemployed have higher death rate – study shows'.

The third piece of research to emerge during 1982 which was to have an important impact on the debate was carried out in Scotland. It was a study by Steve Platt of the Medical Research

Council's Psychiatric Epidemiology Unit in Edinburgh of the relationship between parasuicide ('attempted suicide') and unemployment. Unlike the others, it was reported in the media before the publication of a paper in an academic journal. Platt had spoken to a journalist from BBC Radio's 'Reporting Scotland' looking for expert briefing from his unit more or less as a matter of routine. His comments were reported on 12 August in the *Glasgow Herald* ('Study links suicide with unemployment') and on 13 August in the *Scottish Daily Express* ('A job to survive'). A short version of a literature review in the course of being written for an academic journal (Platt 1984b) of the evidence relating unemployment to suicide was published in the *Unemployment Unit Bulletin* in November of the same year (Platt 1982). The paper made no claims that unemployment necessarily exerted a 'causal' effect on suicide, but stated rather that the evidence so far suggested the risk of both unemployment and suicide are elevated by the presence of psychiatric illness (especially depression), rather than that unemployment is an immediate cause of suicide (Platt 1982).

These findings were all cautiously presented, and due to the way in which they had been arrived at, by making opportunistic use of studies not designed to investigate the effect of unemployment on health specifically, the credibility of the findings was relatively open to attack. Members of all three research groups were stimulated by finding themselves in a position to take part in a high-profile debate, and to tackle what seemed to be a question of importance in both academic and political terms. But this kind of research alone could do little more than produce further twists in the 'loop' of claim and counterclaim. During the summer of 1982, another paper appeared putting the other side of the story: Jon Stern's 'Does unemployment really kill?', was published, coincidentally, it seems, in *New Society* the day after the OPCS LS, 10 June (pp. 421–2). Stern noted that groups of people, whether socially or geographically defined, with high rates of unemployment, are consistently found to have high rates of mortality. However, 'the statistical association' he insisted, 'demonstrates nothing at all about cause'. What if the real problem was that the unemployed 'are far more likely to live in depressed areas, to have low incomes, and to live in bad housing conditions when they are in work?' He succinctly summarises the *'ceteris paribus'* question: Given that a lot of unemployment is concentrated among groups who have high mortality rates anyway, one must also allow for ill-health – physical or mental – causing un-employment and/or causing people to remain unemployed for long periods.

Stern argued in this paper, as he and his colleagues had in their earlier *Lancet* paper, that the reason Brenner's time-series had obtained results strongly suggesting a causal relationship between unemployment rates and mortality rates for the period 1926–76 was the massive social change which occurred roughly in the middle of this period which included the introduction of the welfare state in Britain. Stern enumerates specifically the im-provement in working class diet and medical technology (though they do not mention the near-accomplishment of Beveridge's aim of 'full' employment). He concludes, however, with a personal opinion that unemployment 'does have some effect on health' though this effect has not yet been satisfactorily demonstrated.

Mere associations

During this phase of the debate, arguments for and against an 'effect' began to take an increasingly academic form, less related to proposals for policy change. The issue increasingly emphasised was that of 'association versus causation'. All studies, including the DHSS's own CS had shown that the unemployed were less healthy than the employed. But this did not prove that the rela-tionship was causal. There was no evidence on what happened to men who were known to have been 'healthy' when employed after they lost their jobs. Men in the CS sample already had a relatively high risk of ill health when they entered the study, and did not appear to deteriorate any more if they remained out of the labour force than if they regained work. The LS could say nothing about the health status of its subjects, being derived from infor-mation in the census. Prior to 1991, British censuses contained no question on health. The LS linked census information to death certificates – it could therefore say when people died and what they died from. But it offered no way of knowing what diseases or disabilities they might have experienced during life. Unlike the CS the LS could not give any estimation of the length of spells of unemployment: men described as 'the unemployed' were those who said they were 'seeking work' in the week before the 1971 Census. This group would have included men who had just been made redundant, at one extreme, and very long term unem-ployed at the other. The point made by Stern was that those who experience more unemployment are more likely to appear as 'unemployed' in surveys. This is for the simple but sometimes overlooked reason that the more days one is unemployed, the more likely it is that a survey will take place on one of those days. So that whatever effects are shown by long term follow-up of such a group will be biased towards the consequences of long term or frequent unemployment. Platt's work, as admitted by the author, could be showing a relationship between mental instability and both job loss and suicidal behaviour.

The 'loop' of academic argument had a damping effect on the activity of pressure groups. There seemed to be no answer to the problem of whether men became unemployed because of their health because there were no studies which had examined the health of men before they became unemployed. Members of SCUF reported themselves somewhat demoralised by Jon Stern's address to their September 1981 meeting (along the lines of his 1982 paper in *New Society*), which a founder member recalled as 'crushing'. The first meeting of 1982, on 6 January, was only attended by five people, and by March of 1983 this group had stopped meeting altogether, for reasons which participants were not fully able to explain, but seem to have been dominated by pressure of work on two of its leading members who both took up new posts during the period.

In the summer attendance at meetings of the Liverpool-based UHSG was also falling off and discussion on the role of the group began to be felt necessary. At the July meeting Steve Watkins, a community physician, raised the possibility of a 'North Western Unemployment Alliance' aiming to enrol pressure groups for the unemployed and trade unions. Having by now read the Regional Heart Study paper and the relevant bits of the OPCS LS monograph, he told the group that 'the causal link between unemployment and health could be confidently upheld' nevertheless and felt it was 'important that people should realise this, that DHSS and political interests ... should appreciate that scientific evidence was now available to disprove the claims based on the inadequate and unscientific DHSS Cohort Study.'

The authors of the 'more scientific' papers from the Edinburgh Unit, the Regional Heart Study or LS would probably not have placed themselves in such sharp opposition to the CS at this stage. Neither paper made claims to have demonstrated either that raised morbidity or mortality in the unemployed was not due to

class position, behaviour or 'personal characteristics', let alone
that there was a causal link. Neither were the authors of the CS
eager to place too much weight on their findings. The study, it
was repeatedly pointed out, was not designed to investigate
health. As one put it: 'The incorporation of health questions ...
was a late "tack-on" by which the Department could "do something" about the employment and health issue at minimum cost.
There were always concerns about whether these questions
would be at all useful'.

Discussion at meetings of the UHSG showed no awareness of
the ambivalence of research professionals and academic advisers
to the CS. In addition, throughout the period from late 1981 to the
end of 1982, there seemed to be no awareness of the most important 'behind-the-scenes-activity' going on at the DHSS Headquarters at Elephant and Castle. Had they operated in the way
Whitely and Winyard (1983, 1984) describe other types of pressure groups, keeping in close touch with actual or potential sympathisers *within* relevant government departments, they could
hardly have failed to become aware of developments. As it was,
the group regarded 'the DHSS', because of the role played by
Ramsden and Smee's paper in the controversy over Brenner's
work, as monolithic and hostile. Their one point of regular contact
with the Department was to send copies of their minutes to an
administrator, John Middleton – sometimes in a somewhat modi-
fied form for strategic reasons.

What they might have discovered was that there was more
sympathetic curiosity about whether unemployment affected
health inside the Department than was being publicly indicated
by press releases and Ministerial speeches. Middleton was a
member of a small policy unit called PSU (Policy Strategy Unit)
which had been set up within the DHSS in 1980, on the model of a
mini-think-tank. The PSU existed from 1980 to 1984, and in a
volume of *Minutes of Evidence to the Social Services Select Committee*
(1981, p. 2) was described thus:

> the policy planning unit [of the Community Services Divi-
> sion of the DHSS] has been replaced by the Policy Strategy
> Unit, headed by an assistant secretary and composed of
> three full-time principals and three part-time professional
> staff. It is charged to maintain an overview of policy work in
> all parts of the Department, preparing periodic review of
> policy initiatives and identifying all apparent gaps (particu-

larly of a cross-sector character). It will also receive papers on all major policy reviews within or involving the Department, and is expected to comment from the angle of wider and future policy considerations. Additionally, the unit will carry out specific policy studies or reviews, mainly but not always short-term.

On 14 October 1981, Jack Barnes, a senior member of PSU, was present at a meeting in Prof Walter Holland's Department of Community Medicine at St Thomas's Hospital Medical School (also present were Alwyn Smith, an early member of the UHSG, Stephen Farrow, Steve Engelman and a representative from the Regional Heart Study). It had been called to see what light the combined forces of community medicine and epidemiology might be able to throw on the effect of unemployment on health. Much of the work of the St Thomas' department is funded by the DHSS, which makes it possible that this meeting was a PSU initiative. Partly as a result of these deliberations, on 14 July 1982, a proposal was submitted to the Health Services Research Committee of the Scottish Home and Health Department by two health economists, Steve Engelman of Edinburgh and John Forbes of Glasgow, and from there passed on to the DHSS.

Forbes and Engleman could see that in order to get round the objection that much of the existing research could not show whether unemployment or ill health came first, a longitudinal study including both employed and unemployed was necessary. In their opinion, the one longitudinal study in the field, the OPCS one, was not able to answer this question because the Census does not ask people about their state of health. So that people unemployed at the Census might have been in poorer health as well, and this might be the cause of their unemployment. Their proposal was for a large, three-year cohort study with a projected cost of £120,000 which in their judgement was the only way to get any further.

In September 1982, DHSS officials involved in the work of the PSU submitted a proposal based on the Edinburgh design to Ministers with a positive recommendation. They justified this preference on both academic and political grounds: senior administrators cautioned that anything less would be seen by MPs as a 'low-key response'. The Department of Employment was thought to be about to publish a report on 'Social and other aspects (including health) of unemployment' which 'was not likely to be reassuring'. Ministers were warned to expect fireworks in Parliament, and it was suggested to them by officials that they would 'want to have a line agreed' on unemployment and health by the next session. The seriousness of the issue seemed to justify a large longitudinal study as 'anything else would be hard to justify in the House'. Other studies, smaller in scale, might be useful (these officials admitted) to 'promote good practice' by health authorities, however, any discussions on job creation might risk 'stepping on the toes of the Department of Employment or MSC', something to be strictly avoided.

By early November of 1982, officials in the PSU and the DHSS Chief Scientist's Office were already in the position of having to try and change the minds of the two unsympathetic health ministers, Geoffrey Finsberg and Kenneth Clarke. 'Crudely' one official later remarked, 'the Minister didn't want to know.' Kenneth Clarke had been willing to admit that unemployment was a bad thing. The answer was, therefore, to create more real jobs, which was what government policy had consistently attempted to do in any case. The civil servants protested that the Health and Personal Social Services side of DHSS had a duty to see whether there were measures it should take to mitigate specific health effects of unemployment, and justified their persistent desire for research to proceed on these practical grounds. Different measures might be needed according to whether ill health was a cause or consequence of unemployment, and only the long-term study of the problem could answer that question. Their appeals were unsuccessful. The proposal ended up in a DHSS file (where it lay as late as 1986) as having been 'deferred pending consideration of resources', with an attached proposal for joint funding by the English, Welsh and Scottish Health Departments, the Department of Employment and the research councils.

On 17 January 1983, Ernie Ross, MP for Dundee (West), asked the Secretary of State for Scotland 'what evidence he has that infant mortality rates amongst unemployed families are greater than amongst employed families', and 'if the Secretary of State was sponsoring any research projects into the effects of unemployment upon health in Scotland' (*Hansard* 25 January WA col. 37) Under-Secretary of State for Scotland John Mackay replied: 'My department is not funding any research projects directly related to the effects of unemployment upon health in Scotland'. On 25 January, Ross followed-up by demands that the Secretary of State for Scotland seek to fund research projects related to the effects of unemployment upon health in Scotland (*Hansard* 25 January WA col. 423). At this time, Mackay responded: 'My Department has under consideration an application for funding of a research project related to unemployment and health.' What may have happened here is that after the decision of November 1982 not to provide DHSS funds for a project based on Forbes and Engelman's proposal, the Scottish Home and Health Department gave some consideration to funding a more limited project. No one interviewed in Scotland in the spring and summer of 1983 mentioned any further applications subsequent to the rejection of Forbes and Engelman's. However after the decision of November 1982, DHSS funding looked extremely unlikely. Forbes remembers getting a letter finally turning down the proposal 'sometime after the [1983] general election'. In the event, Mackay's answer seems to have satisfied the Scottish MPs for the time being, as the Adjournment Debate on Unemployment in Scotland introduced by John Maxton on 8 February contained no references to health at all.

None of this was reflected in the recorded discussion of the members of the UHSG, either at the end of 1982, throughout 1983, nor indeed as late as 1986. Steve Watkins commented that UHSG had not really been set up as a 'pressure group' at all, but more as what its title implies – a study group – to support his own research in community medicine and that of other members of the group. (In a similar career move to that taken by Len Fagin, Watkins had undertaken a project on health and economic change as part of his registrarship.) In 1982, he felt, looking back, the group's meetings had become 'stereotyped meetings that had lost their point.' It had kept going partly because there was a demand for information and speakers (as SCUF had also found), and because his own work and that of his colleagues still needed a forum for discussion. Although the initiative to convene a North-Western Unemployment Alliance came to nothing, it marks the place at which the ideas of the 'study group' turned away from 'research' and towards 'policy'.

Policy and strategy

At the end of November, a Marplan poll carried out for the *Guardian* showed that 'a mood of fatalism' had settled over Britain, whereby seven out of ten voters thought unemployment the dominant political issue, but few thought there was any solution on offer by opposition political parties. Ten times as many people cited unemployment as 'the main problem' as those who cited inflation, with law and order taking second place. This 'mood of the country' may be considered one reason why the new research on unemployment and health had so little impact. Journalists were aware of it, and felt that people did not want to 'have their noses rubbed' in what seemed an irremediable fact of life. Another reason for the low public profile of the research on health and unemployment may have been that at this time it was not the policy of the Medical Research Council, which was funding a high proportion of the relevant work, to encourage its staff to offer 'information subsidies' to the media (though by early 1986, under pressure of cuts in research council funding, it had appointed a Press Officer). The LS monograph in particular was too long and complicated to be digestible by the media, and no pressure group had, as yet, produced anything suitably pre-digested. Some members of the LS and British Regional Heart Study teams were somewhat disappointed by the lack of impact of their work. They had, at that time, little idea of 'information subsidy' or of how the media work, and rather expected journalists to contact them enthusiastically, having read their work in the learned journals. Only poor scientists, they felt, needed to engage in deliberate 'soapbox' exercises.

From 1982 onwards, in terms of 'public opinion', unemployment came to hold a somewhat paradoxical position. From available evidence, it seems that unemployment was both acknowledged as the biggest 'social problem' in British society, and that it was decreasingly regarded as something which could strike at anyone. For the majority of people, therefore, to be worried about unemployment came to be seen as a disinterested moral concern rather than an immediate worry. These tendencies were confirmed in a survey carried out in 1986 (Linton 1987) which showed wide contrast in the issues which respondents saw as 'important to the nation as a whole' and 'important to them as individuals'. In terms of labour economics, these shifts in public attitude were well founded upon the tendency of the British labour market to become more segmented as unemployment stabilised at a higher level, after the rapid rise of 1981. As unemployment became less a mischance that could befall anyone, possible health consequences seemed to become less of a public and more of a professional issue.

Notes

1. A similar exercise was carried out by the General Register Office, Scotland, but data on unemployment and health were never analysed, presumably because this would have been a much smaller study.
2. It should be noted here that the article in *The Times* more or less allows readers to define for themselves what is meant by 'the unemployed'. In fact, 'unemployment' in this study is operationalised as ' "seeking work" in the week before Census night 1971'.

5
BREAKING THE LOOP

Making the papers

Some of the ambivalence of the atmosphere in which the debate now proceeed, and the sheer contingency of some of the processes involved, may be seen by close examination of the way in which unemployment and parasuicide made its next major appearance in the media. On 13 March 1983, Steve Platt gave a talk on youth and drugs at Moray House College of Education in Edinburgh. A *Scotsman* reporter, Bryan Christie covered the event as part of his routine work – tasks are allocated to reporters at the beginning of a working shift, and this one happened to fall to him. He reported it on 14 March, but this was not the end of the matter. As it happened, Christie (who later became health correspondent of *The Scotsman)* had ambitions to be a feature writer, was interested in health issues, and *The Scotsman* had no one else writing on health at this time. As Christie described events:

> It was just an off chance. He [Platt] said he hadn't finished the research yet, so I left it for a while, and then phoned him and said how's it going? He said he was writing it up so I left it a few more weeks. I was looking for things to write features about ... The trouble is, if you follow up something like this, you still have to do all the other stuff as well, all the routine reporting.

Nevertheless, Steve Platt felt that Christie dealt with the issue (in a feature which appeared on 2 August 1983) with great care and accuracy. The article acknowledges that a 'significant relationship' does not amount to a 'causal link'. However, Christie quoted Platt:

> The trouble with this area of research is that it is very con- tentious and the academic community have in the past sat on the fence. They have felt for too long that they have to dot the i's and cross the t's but it can now be said that the risks associated with long-term unemployment are just not acceptable.'

Combining the requirements of 'reporter' with those of 'science writer', Christie added other items to his summary of the work on parasuicide: a 'human-interest story' about two young men who suffocated themselves, leaving a note saying they had 'nothing to live for', parliamentary questions, and ministerial denials.

In common with other Scottish journalists whom I interviewed, Christie bemoaned the way in which the organisation of work and limitation of resources on a small newspaper made it difficult to deal with issues in depth. As he put it later:

> I can understand that the journalistic profession is not re-nowned for treating things like this with care. It is very easy to read the figures wrong. If you're handed something on a piece of paper at five thirty and told you've got half an hour to work on it, mistakes do happen.

and his colleague on *The Scotsman*, Robbie Dinwoodie, remarked:

> You have to understand ... there are only nine reporters on *The Scotsman*. So ... journalism becomes a reactive business. If someone doesn't come to tell you about something [that happens in a scientific debate], you'll never find out about it. It's fire-brigade journalism.

To add to the difficulties, Christie had other strong interests apart from health at this time, for example, in defence issues. His colleague Sarah Nelson, who also wrote some features on health and medicine, was soon offered (and accepted) the specialised post of education correspondent, a particularly important topic in Scotland. Not only for unemployment and health, but for any technically complicated issue, lack of a specialist writer was a serious problem. In the case of *The Scotsman*, quality did not suffer, but quantity may have.

Christie concluded his 2 August feature in eloquent Calvinist vein: 'Work, it has been said, is nature's physician ...' He admitted later, however, that there had been no letters to the newspaper following his feature, and that he had been 'surprised at how quickly it went flat'. By the time Steve Platt felt ready to discuss his work, Parliament had gone into recess, so that it had been

> hard to find people to chase up for comments on it. It was hard enough work trying to make sure I got all the figures right ... I phoned the Press Office at the SHHD and tried to arrange a meeting with MacKay. Of course he wasn't going to have any of that.

The 'World at One' did follow up the article, but no other Scottish newspaper did, not even the Edinburgh *Evening News*, which shares premises with *The Scotsman* and has a good local reputation for covering medicine and health On 4 August *The Daily Telegraph* carried a very small piece and the *Morning Star* gave the story rather more space ('Joblessness kills, shock probe reveals').

At around the same time, the regular bulletin reporting the doings of MRC researchers, *MRC News* carried a long discussion of Platt's work, and this was reported in the *Daily Star* as:

> Doctors are shocked by a huge increase in suicide attempts by the unemployed ... the Medical Research Council says there is 'cause for alarm'.

This somewhat sensational-sounding phrase, 'cause for alarm', is in fact a direct quote from *MRC Bulletin No. 20*. It provides an example of the fine line to be trodden between the scientific entrepreneurialism necessary to keep a researchable social problem sufficiently in the limelight and not giving grist to the mill of sensationalism. The report in *MRC News* cautions that the existence of the association demonstrated by Platt's work does not 'constitute proof of a causal link', and then goes on to state that 'a causal explanation appears more likely'.

In November of 1983 Steve Platt's research on unemployment and parasuicide was published in the *Unemployment Unit Bulletin*. Like the report of his work in *MRC News*, this paper stresses the 'public health' aspect of the problem:

> Clearly, far more research remains to be carried out in this area. It should have high priority ... because of its practical, public health implications. If trends in long-term unemployment are indeed crucial for predicting the future course of parasuicide, then there is grave cause for alarm ... Whatever the nature of the association between unemployment and parasuicide, it has been shown that [the] long-term jobless currently run more than 18 times the risk of parasuicide of the employed. (Platt 1983)

and the proposed solution:

> This ... risk may be reduced to some extent by allocating more resources to help alleviate the economic, psychological and social impact of prolonged joblessness ... But ... these measures do not address the fundamental underlying problem ... Urgent government action is required to reduce the level of unemployment. (*Unemployment Unit Bulletin*, November 1983. no. 10, pp. 4–5)

Surprisingly, *The Scotsman* carried no report of this publication. The Unemployment Unit was experienced in the art of information subsidy as practised in England, and had provided copies of the *Unemployment Unit Bulletin* to all national newspapers' head offices. Many did carry the story. The editor of *The Scotsman* decided not to carry another article as it was too soon after the August one. Bryan Christie was on holiday. When he returned he was dismayed at his editor's decision. To add insult to injury, the *Glasgow Herald* had covered the story. As he put it:

> Not many people read both the *Glasgow Herald* and *The Scotsman*, except for journalists, that is! But if they had, it would have looked as if the *Herald* had got a good story and we had missed it altogether. At the very least, we could have pointed out that we covered it months ago ... We could have pointed out that we had beaten the *Glasgow Herald*.

In fact, the article received wider coverage in English newspapers than in Scottish ones, which puzzled Steve Platt. This was a result of the Unemployment Unit's unfamiliarity with the ways in which the media deal with Scottish issues. The *Daily Mail* contacted Platt from London after reading the story in the *Glasgow Herald*. Why was this necessary when copies of the Bulletin had been sent to the *Mail's* London HQ? The right thing to have done, explained Bryan Christie, was to have sent it to the *Mail's* Scottish HQ. Otherwise, if they decided it was not a 'British' issue, London would not bother to notify the *Mail's* Scottish offices in Glasgow. If one had wanted to get coverage in the Scottish *Daily Express*, just to complicate matters further, the best thing would be to send press notices to the *Express's* Manchester offices, where their Scottish news desk is located. 'It all depends,' he pointed out, 'what you mean by a national newspaper.'

This account of how one piece of research 'made the papers' shows the operation of an 'accident-prone process' by which scientific findings reach the wider public (as shown in Chapter 2 for 'World in Action's' coverage of Brenner's claims). It also provides an example of how a researcher's participation in one social-problem process (on drugs) can lead to the adoption of an 'expert' role in quite a different one.

From research to policy debate: the direct route

As participants in the debate saw it, the loop into which the unemployment and health debate was caught in 1982 and 1983 could be broken by new knowledge. A study designed to provide such knowledge had been submitted for funding and eventually turned down. Although they were not aware of the backstage events surrounding Forbes and Engleman's proposal, members of the UHSG now took a decisive step. They decided to attempt another kind of break-out by addressing the policy debate directly, using such knowledge as was available, despite its controversial nature.

In this 'third stage' of the debate, what is important is not the development of new knowledge claims, but the promotion of value claims more or less regardless of the state of the academic debate. This took the form of a decision to emphasise 'policy' rather than 'research' in the major event of 1983 in the debate, the USHG's 'Policy Workshop', held in Leeds on 24 November. The fairly extensive media coverage of Steve Platt's paper set an appropriate background for the Workshop.

The planning of the Leeds conference provides an example of a group altering its strategy to pursue a new set of alliances, and of the way in which this strategy affected the group's assessment of knowledge-claims. At its first meeting of 1983, congruent with the general tendency throughout the debate for labour movement organisations to be uninterested in 'the health of the unemployed', it was reported that the initiative to set up a North-Western Alliance had met with a very disappointing response ... only two county councils and a single trade union had replied. So the group decided to take over the organisation of what was at first described as a 'national research conference'. This might seem at first to be a turn away from 'politics' towards 'science'. But from the beginning, the purpose of this conference was ambiguous. Steve Watkins remembered it as having been projected as a 'policy conference' but the Group's minutes give a different picture. This ambiguity was to be reflected in the final outcome. At this time full-time professional resarchers had not become involved in the activities of the group. Additionally, their mood, after the heat of the debate between Gravelle *et al.* and Brenner, was cautious. The Regional Heart Study researchers were committed to extreme discretion in the use of their findings, and at least one of the authors of the OPSC LS monograph, at this time, was (at least publicly) far from convinced that the LS results were not due to prior selection of the unemployed by ill health.

At the 24 February meeting of UHSG, there was still no decision as to whether the conference should be on 'policy' or on 're-search'. Members of the study group were usually prepared to be very bold in making claims about the evidence that unemploy-ment caused ill health, but seem to have hesitated over the ques-tion of whether further discussion of 'the evidence' could be done away with altogether. Even by those sympathetically inclined, the debate on whether or not unemployment could be regarded as 'causing' ill health was not at this time regarded as settled. The appearance of new, post-Brenner British research carried out by highly regarded MRC funded teams and using less contentious methods had not made that much difference to the position which any person or group wishing to be seen as 'fair' and 'reasoned', whatever their sympathies, could take.

Of course, while all this was going on, a general election cam-paign was being waged. There is no suggestion, either in UHSG minutes of in interview accounts of what was happening to the group at this time, that the election affected the decisions it took or the plans it made. However, the presence of only three people at the meeting on 21 April may have been partly due to members' other political commitments. At this meeting most time seems to have been devoted to discussion of the proposed conference, or as it now comes to be called, workshop. It was decided to hold it in Leeds in late November, and to deal solely with policy. After-wards, a smaller group of twelve to fifteen people could stay overnight at the Nuffield Centre for Health Service Studies and write a document which the Centre had agreed to produce as an occasional paper. Research papers, were to be solicited, but only as 'background'. By 6 July, the Study Group had decided (at a meeting of still only three people) that precirculated research papers would only prove diversionary. So brief summary papers were to be requested, from Watkins on physical health, Platt on suicide and parasuicide, and a leading expert on the effect of unemployment on physical health, Prof Peter Warr of Sheffield University on general mental health effects.

The ambiguity of the group's discussion leading up to the conference was reflected on the day, in an uneasy opening discus-sion which hovered constantly on the brink of the discouraged re-evaluation of 'research'. Steve Watkins, author of a position-paper circulated prior to the conference which made very sweep-ing claims in favour of a 'pro-Brenner' position, at one point admitted that 'It is still not clear just what it is that is important for

health about work.' And Scott-Samuel reminded the meeting that
'A minister in the House of Commons can get up and say there
are no proven links. They are still able to do this, though I don't
know how they can after the evidence of the Longitudinal Study'.

Composition of the Leeds Policy Seminar	
'Activists'	12
(local councillors, trade unionists, local action groups)	
'Academics'	17
of which: Economists	2
Psychologists	4
Sociologists	11
Community physicians	6
GPs	1
Local authority employees	3
Health Educators	6
Total	45

The scope of possible alliances for Manifesto community medicine is visible here: academics from various disciplines, health
educators, and 'activists' of various kinds, all groups which were
also represented by papers published in the 'official' journal *Community Medicine* as well as its 'Radical' doppleganger.

One community physician offered an interesting view of the
relationship between research and policy in this and other debates when he observed that: 'Those involved in research find it
difficult to at the same time be questioning about the limits of the
state of knowledge and also to say,in a policy-making sense, "we
can regard this as fact".' Academic social scientists (leaving aside
psychologists for the moment), did not confine themselves to
research and its application, but also made more openly political
contributions. However, in general their interventions in the discussion reflected concerns with their relationship to the state: 'It is
increasingly obvious to me that the response of the state is ...
always an attempt to refute these studies [such as Brenner and the
Longitudinal Study]. That's the way it was in the 1930s and that's
the way it is now.'

Thoughts on the media were:

>   Part of the problem is in the timidity of researchers about
>   their own results ... We cannot *prove* the connection in the
>   same way as a randomized controlled trial can. You have to
>   educate people in the media that this kind of research is not
>   'inferior' to natural-scientific research.

Community workers and 'activists' (delegates from Labour
Parties, Trade Union research departments, action goups, etc.)
debated the relative merits of attempting to change national
macro-economic policy versus those of encouraging local initiatives, though on the whole these participants were not particularly vocal, and a solution to the central-local conflict was offered
by an academic who was also involved in political initiatives at
both levels:

>   there seem to be two perspectives among health workers:
>   The first is, 'we don't want to get involved in unemploy-
>   ment ... it's too political'. Others take the attitude that the
>   response is ameliorative ,not political enough. One way to
>   meet these objections is not to separate prevention and
>   modification of effects. If people get involved in preventive
>   work, it may help to transform their attitude to unemploy-
>   ment on the wider political level.

There were two groups who contributed fairly extensively to
the general discussion in this meeting, but which did not enter the
alliance which gave much of its shape to the rest of the debate on
the health of the unemployed. These were the psychologists and
what I will call the 'futurologists' that is, economists and other
social scientists engaged in the study of long-range economic and
scientific policy and planning. They tended to take a pessimistic
view and to see growing numbers of unemployed as an inevitable
result of technological progress. One 'futurologist' Ian Miles of
Sussex University's Science Policy Research Unit, felt that as a
result, efforts should be turned towards finding other ways of
providing the health-protective features of work: 'We need to talk
about restructuring society so as to provide more opportunities
for people to exercise control over their 'everyday lives, to become
involved in social networks, and constructive activities'.

The contribution of the psychologists was perhaps most sober-
ing of all. They accepted the prediction of the 'futurologists' and
saw the task of local educators and service providers to be one
of countering the 'work ethic'. Steve McKenna from the same
research unit in Sheffield as Peter Warr (who did not attend)

pointed out that 20 per cent of people in their studies experienced improvements in physical health after redundancies or during periods of lay-off from heavy jobs such as shipbuilding. He also felt that: 'The will to work is diminishing. We should think about how we are training schoolkids to demand work. We're turning out people with a high employment commitment which cannot be satisfied'.

And a clinical psychologist, Graham Stokes asked:

When we talk about local campaigns, what is our focus? Should we not acknowledge that technology is changing and a lot of people will never get paid employment again? Even if we got back to the level of production of the 1970s, in the West Midlands, the effect on employment would be minimal, because of changes in technology and higher productivity.

It can be seen from these extracts from the day's discussions that not all of what the psychologists and 'futurologists' were offering could have been easily incorporated into the line of argument being developed at that time by the UHSG's leadership. Their contributions were in line with the sort of thinking that lay behind Len Fagin's research: that unemployment was a stigmatising condition which offered few opportunities for psychological resolution of bereavement and loss. Policy prescriptions following from this included notions of re-orienting young people's aspirations away from work altogether. This ran against the grain of what others concerned with social policies wished to argue – that government policy must change in a Keynesian direction towards the goal of full employment. Although less directly challenging in political terms, the 'futurologists' recommendations would not, presumably, have been particularly tempting to monetarists, who saw high unemployment as a method for curbing inflation by lowering wage claims. If the unemployed were to accept their state more easily, the incentive to undercut those still in work would presumably be decreased. Although Miles and Stokes continued to publish work on the subject of the health (particularly mental health) of unemployed people, this did not enter the main stream of either political or academic debate.

But the importance of the meeting was the atttempt to break out of the loop of evidence and counter-evidence by a self-conscious decision (infuriating even to some of its sympathisers) to treat the evidence they had as if it were sufficient to get on with policy prescription. The product of the workshop was the report 'Unemployment, health and social policy'. Specific policy measures advocated in the report did not only emphasise economic measures to increase employment, however. It major recommendations were:

- improved levels of benefits;
- free public transport and recreation facilities for unemployed people;
- job creation;
- voluntary and flexible early retirement policies;
- work sharing and shorter hours of work;
- avoidance of psychological damage to unemployed people through stigma; and
- encouragement of support groups.

As previously agreed, the Nuffield Centre for Health Services Studies financed the publication of the report, but it did not appear for almost a year.

January 1984: The status of the debate

Following the decision by the pressure group, and some other participants, to take the initiative regardless of whether or not the academic debate need be regarded as 'settled', some of the 'experts' themselves now began to play a more active role; 1984 began with the swansong of the USHP. Its original Kings Fund money had run from 1975–80, and was then replaced by a grant from the Health Education Council, and others for specific projects from the Leverhulme Foundation (1980–83) and the Rowntree Trust (1981–March 1984). By the end of 1983, most USHP staff were looking for or had found other jobs.

On 19 January 1984, *New Society* feature writer Martyn Harris summed up the 'state of the art' in unemployment and health research as far as non-expert but informed opinion may have seen it at this time (Harris 1984). Harris reminded his readers that while the average two-child family spent £124.75 per week excluding housing costs in 1981, the current (1983) rate of Supplementary Benefit for such a family was £59.20 per week, around 40 per cent of the amount *spent* (not *earned*) by a family with an employed breadwinner. Under a subheading 'The problem of proof' he described the 'loop' in which the debate on health was now caught. Work by Len Fagin was described as not 'particularly rigorous or exhaustive'. He regarded Brenner's work as 'The most

powerful argument for a causal link between unemployment and
health' and reported that although Brenner's results 'not surprisingly ... have been savagely attacked' nevertheless 'they appear
to be standing up fairly well, with many social scientists paying
respectful attention to his findings, if only because they don't
understand how he obtained them.' On mental health, Harris
reported, there was agreement, except for suicide and attempted
suicide, and here he quoted Steve Platt's work, which demonstrated Platt and the Unemployment Unit's success in producing
the November 1983 information subsidy. He comments also on
the relative 'lack of interest' in unemployment and health in the
1980s in comparison to the 1930s. In his final paragraph, using
rather strong phrases, he asked:

> Is it that the social science establishment has actually col-
> lapsed under the steady sniping from the Keith Joseph quar-
> ter and lacks the self-confidence to tackle the major social
> issue of the day ... It is a bit difficult to argue for the defence
> of benefits and services if you can't even establish the true
> costs of unemployment to the hatchet men in Whitehall.
> (Harris 1984)

In this final paragraph, Harris foreshadows the way in which
the media, at least, will now begin to deal with the unemployment and health issue. No longer as a 'social problem' in its own
right, but as *just one* indicator of two other 'social problems', now
more interesting and relevant to the media, and, importantly,
shared by media workers, government scientific advisers, and
other academics and scientists. One of these new 'problems' was
the decline in the volume, availability and intelligibility of officially produced and available information on 'social indicators'.
This was not only a problem for journalists, (who, as has been
explained, need information not just in any form, but preferably
in a 'subsidized' form), but also for research and policy units
within government departments, in the wake of the Rayner reviews and changes in the organisation and funding of official
surveys.[1] The second 'problem' was the 'decline in British science'
(especially social science). For participants in the unemployment
and health debate, this came closest to home in the form of the
review by Lord Rothschild of the working of the Social Science
Research Council initiated by Sir Keith Joseph, as reflected in the
above quote from Martyn Harris' article. The review was widely
seen as a prelude to cuts in funding for social science. In the event,

the recommendations of Lord Rothschild's report (Rothschild 1982) were far more benign (Posner 1982), although in its aftermath the Council lost the word 'science' from its name.[2] A new alliance then began to take shape, between researchers both inside and outside government on the one hand, and journalists on the 'quality' papers on the other. Academic advisers to government departments as well as some professional civil servants appear to have been increasingly willing to talk off the record to journalists. Interviewed for this study (in early 1986), a senior medical academic gave the opinion that:

> the really interesting story [concerning unemployment and health in Britain] is why the research in Britain *is* so thin … [but] this could not be investigated by an academic, but would have to be left to investigative journalism. If you tell a journalist something, the more confidential you say it is, the more certain he is to print it … But as an academic, you [the interviewer] cannot betray those confidences. After all, these people [academics] have to go on trying to get funded by this blessed government. It is a question of the best being the enemy of the good.

In this quote, the speaker also gives his perception of how the debate might have been affected by 'political context', in that he clearly believes research funds would have been easier to come by under a government of a different complexion.

Point of passage

It was in this context in mid-1984 that the results of analysing the ten-year mortality data from the OPCS LS first became available, and began to be presented as fresh support for the claims that 'unemployment harms health'. In this second phase of their work on unemployment, the LS team began to tackle the *ceteris paribus* question head on. Were some people selected into unemployment because they were in poor health in the first place? Could any of the limited number of studies in a position to produce evidence on the issue throw any light on this question?

The first full account of the ten-year follow-up results of the LS were given in a talk by Dr David Jones, a senior research fellow working with John Fox at the Social Statistics Research Unit at City University. The occasion was a conference of the Institute of Statisticians at Kent University in July 1984. One half-day of the conference was devoted to the topic of unemployment and health.

The rest of the conference, on 'health statistics' was, however, dominated by topics of interest either to planners or drug companies. Perhaps as a result of this, the session on unemployment was poorly attended.

Derek Cook of the British Regional Heart Study team gave the first paper in the session, in effect repeating most of the material in a review paper which he had written for an edited collection of *Recent Advances in Occupational Health* (Cook 1985, Cook and Shaper 1985). For the purposes of this public presentation, however, he emphasised the dramatic nature of the public debate, starting with a slide which showed a collage of headlines representing both 'sides' of the debate: 'Death on the dole'; 'A scandal on the conscience of Margaret Thatcher'; 'Dole is like a holiday, says economist'. He also reminded his audience that: 'The funding of research is a political matter. It is futile to pretend that we can deal with such a topic in a purely objective way'.

In this and other ways, the tone of this paper was very different from that of the review. Cook laid more emphasis on the material on nutrition, taken from papers by Cole, Donnet and Stansfield (published in 1983) and by Doyle and co-workers (published in 1982). Cole *et al.* had studied the birthweight and growth of babies in two areas of Glasgow, one prosperous, the other deprived. They had demonstrated lower birthweight in babies whose fathers were unemployed. Doyle *et al.* had studied the diets of pregnant women in two similarly contrasting areas of London. Using the painstaking 'one-week weighed survey' method, they found that pregnant women in the poorer area were consuming under 1,700 calories per day on average, and that these diets were particularly lacking in essential fatty acids necessary for cell-growth, and thus particularly important in pregnancy. That neither of these studies had made any great impact on the public debate was regarded as justified by Cook, in the light of their small size and the fact that they had not been designed to investigate unemployment. He concluded: 'As in the 1930s, national indicators are reassuring, but local studies may tell a different story. I say "may" because I don't think the studies are good enough at present'. However, Cook made no concessions to Brenner, devoting the last section of his talk to an exposition of Gravelle, Stern and Hutchinson's critique ('On the whole, I feel they did succeed in taking his paper apart'). In general, he felt, longitudinal aggregate studies of this nature, which give no data on individuals, could give us no more help in deciding such issues as whether unemployment affected health.

The second speaker, Paul Jackson, a research psychologist at Sheffield University, concentrated on the psychological effects of unemployment. Throughout the debate, psychological effects were regarded as more or less uncontroversial. Accordingly, Jackson's view was that there was 'a consensus on the consequences of unemployment'.

The next paper dealt with the latest result from the OPCS Longitudinal Study, and was based on Working Paper No. 18 from the City University's Social Statistics Research Unit (SSRU). Although the first author of this and of all subsequent papers on unemployment and health was Kath Moser, a research fellow in the SSRU, she disliked giving papers publicly, and as a result a colleague, David Jones was allocated this task. The way in which his talk was constructed was typical of LS 'style'. He began by setting out three alternative hypotheses about the relationship between unemployment and health:

Model 1. That unemployment has an adverse effect on health

$$U \longrightarrow H$$

Model 2. That unhealthy people are either

a. more likely to be unemployed or
b. at a higher risk of death [so that it is their ill health which 'causes' BOTH the unemployment AND the mortality.]

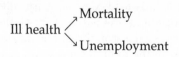

Model 3. That there are other factors associated with both unemployment and an increased risk of mortality (which '... might be social disadvantage')

$$\text{(Other factor)} \begin{cases} \nearrow U \\ \searrow M \end{cases}$$

(Where: U = unemployment; H = health and M = mortality)

Table 5.1 Numbers at risk and crude death rates: men seeking work at 1971 census.

	At risk 1971	Died 1971-81	Crude death rate
All men	250,588	29,923	11.94%
15–65	161,699	8,061	5.0%
seeking work	5,861	328	5.6%

(i.e. those 'seeking work' were approximately 12% more likely to die in the following ten year period than all men in the sample aged 15–65)
The unemployment rate was 3.6% in 1971.

Table 5.1. shows the basic numbers on which the findings are based. It is notable that the number of men 'seeking work' in the week before census night 1971 who died between 1971 and 1981 was only 328. In longitudinal studies, death rates are not calculated in the 'crude' manner used in the above table, but by a somewhat more complex method which makes use of the concept of 'person-years at risk'. The basic idea behind this method is to establish the denominator used to calculate the *rate* of (say) death taking account of the fact that as people die the size of the population at risk changes. The investigator cannot simply count up all the deaths by the end of the period of study and divide that by the number of people at the beginning. Having carried out this correction, mortality must then be standardised to take account of the possibility that the ages of unemployed people may be different from those of the employed. Otherwise an apparent excess could be merely the result of an age difference between the two groups. This gives a measures known as a Standardised Mortality Ratio or SMR. The SMR for those seeking work in 1971 was, according to age (see Table 5.2).

Table 5.2 Standardised mortality ratio by age, 1971.

Men 'seeking work' 1971 SMR (Average=100)		95% confidence limits
15–24	169	ALL
25–34	178	
35–44	201	VERY
4554	173	
55–64	111	LARGE

Table 5.3 Social class distribution of the 'seeking work'

Social Class	% Seeking Work					
	I	II	IIIn	IIIm	IV	V
Ut. rate	1.2	1.8	2.1	2.9	3.9	8.6

Table 5.4 SMR for those 'seeking work' in different social classes

Class	I	II	IIIn	IIIm	IV	V
SMR	103	139	116	132	150	124

David Jones then presented the first of the arguments, that the overall mortality excess of 36 per cent in the 'unemployed' was due to their social class distribution. Unemployment is more common in manual than non manual classes, and a great deal more common in social class V (unskilled) (see Table 5.3). So a further correction or 'standardisation' had to be carried out to allow for this (see Table 5.4).

Table 5.4 shows that mortality is raised in men of all social classes. Social class standardisation did reduce the overall excess mortality of unemployed men in the sample from 36 per cent to 21 per cent. However, Jones then pointed out that when the unemployed men whose usual occupation was 'inadequately described' (those with inadequately described occupations had an unemployment rate of 50.6 per cent) were removed from the analysis, the excess mortality adjusted for social class was 33 per cent (i.e. SMR 133), a much smaller effect of standardisation. On standardisation for housing tenure, a variable which the LS team regarded as a good measure of social position, the excess was also reduced, to 27 per cent. From this Jones concluded that '*some* of the mortality in the unemployed may be accounted for by their distribution by social class.' He next asked, was there a 'reverse effect' which had been strongly proposed by Derek Cook in his paper, whereby those already in poor health were selected into unemployment?

At this point Jones introduced, for the first time in a public report of LS results, the concept of 'the wearing-off of selection' although he does not use this term. This concept was to play an important role in the rest of the debate. As he put it:

Is there a health related selection effect? If that were the case, we'd expect the mortality rate to fall off with time, as the unhealthy subset died off. We'd expect the fall to be much more marked in the acute diseases, as well. In fact, what we find is that for all-causes there is [over time] an *increase*, not a decrease in the excess mortality associated with unemployment. Suicide does not decrease at all. Lung cancer does show a larger fall, but bronchitis and emphysema ... do not. This is because *the very sick have died.*

In this passage can be seen the emergence into the unemployment and health debate of the intricate argument about how to test for 'selective effects' when using data from longitudinal studies, first set out in the monograph which gave the first results of the main LS analysis (Fox and Goldblatt 1982, and for some discussion see Bartley 1991). The LS team were proposing that the problem of not knowing what state of health people were in before they became unemployed could be solved without new studies. If the excess mortality in the unemployed decreases over time, then there is evidence that the unemployed were ill in the first place. As this is not found, the evidence goes the other way. Jones concluded this section of his talk by observing that his figures could not be regarded as providing 'strong corroboration of the view that the unemployed have a higher mortality rate because they are sicker in the first place'. This cautious formulation was congruent with the general approach taken to this topic in the study.

Having dealt in this way with both the social class and the health-selection hypotheses, Jones added a new piece of information, on the mortality of wives of men seeking work in 1971. It had been found that these women also experienced higher mortality than that for wives of men in the whole sample, an SMR of 120 for all-causes mortality, which included SMRs of 160 for accidents, violence and suicide, and of 157 for lung cancer. Now, whereas it might still be that somehow or other, men were selected into 'unemployment' by ill health, it did not seem at all plausible that women would somehow be selected into marriage with 'potentially unemployed' men by similar criteria (we shall see that this was to be contested but it was not questioned at this meeting). Jones concluded; 'That leaves us with explanation number one, the direct mechanism, if I can call it that.' His overall conclusions were:

- Mortality is raised in those seeking work on Census night 1971.
- Some, but not all, of the excess is attributable to social class, housing tenure, etc.
- Some, but not all, of the remaining excess is explained by a health selection effect.
- Mortality is also raised in other members of the unemployed person's household.
- The residual excess is possibly attributable to unemployment per se.

The key concept in this interpretation of the LS data was the idea that if a difference in mortality between any two groups in a population is caused by some form of 'selection' (represented by the diagram for Model 2 in Jones' talk), then the mortality difference should decrease over time. The 'wearing off of selection' was found extremely difficult to understand by many participants. It was not widely accepted or taken-up by other groups, but rather constituted a barrier to further work, particularly to the work of 'moral fragmentation' which depended on attributing a high level of mortality in a social group to the personal characteristics of group members. There *was* an agreement (tacit rather than explicit) amongst epidemiologists and medical statisticians that consideration of the wearing off of selection effects had to be included in future 'serious' papers on unemployment and health, either to support it or attempt to refute it (though this was ignored by economists, see Forbes and Macgregor 1987). Because few researchers felt able to do this, the 'wearing-off argument' produced the beginnings of another impasse. Even sympathetic groups failed to take it up and use it in pursuit of *their* objectives, and its factual 'solidity' was accordingly fragile. However, a simpler construction of the message of SSRU Working Paper No. 18 was now taken up by the UHSG, and succeeded in once again raising the political profile of 'unemployment and health'.

The balloon goes up again – but not so far this time

By the next meeting of the UHSG, held on 22 August 1984, the report 'Unemployment, health and social policy', (the product of the workshop held in Leeds in November 1983), was being printed. The Manifesto-oriented group of community physicians were perceived (with some resentment) as having written it more or less as they would have intended had the workshop never been held. The opinions of the psychologists and futurologists that young people should be weaned from the work ethic, for example, are conspicuously absent. A publication date was set for 17 September. Meanwhile Scott-Samuel had been sent a copy of the SSRU Working Paper on which David Jones' talk to the Institute of Statisticians had been based. This happened automatically, as his name was on a list (at SSRU) of 'interested persons'. The Study Group had been advised to look for some 'new research findings' with which to link the release of their report, and it looked as if this would serve the purpose very well. After this meeting, Scott-Samuel, on other business in London, found time to speak to both the *Sunday Mirror* and the *Guardian*, in an attempt to associate the Report with the new research in the minds of journalists. The press releases went out embargoed until 16 September, a Sunday, so as to 'catch the Sundays' (attract the attention of the large Sunday newspapers). It described the Study Group as involving 'doctors, policy-makers, academics and unemployed people'. That is, it did *not* concentrate on the 'mainly academic' identity of the group, which in other contexts tended to be emphasised.

In fact, the *Sunday Mirror* of 16 September carried nothing about unemployment and health. Later the editor wrote to Scott-Samuel apologising and explaining that 'Princess Diana's [obstetric] labour problems had usurped the space, but that they planned do something at a later date. Nothing ever appeared in an edition of the *Sunday Mirror*, though later in September the *Daily Mirror* carried a small piece on the Report. On 17 September, the *Guardian* carried a large piece on page 2 which quoted SSRU Working Paper 18 along with a series of estimates made by Scott-Samuel of how many 'unemployment-related deaths had taken place in the year 1984 (Scott-Samuel 1984), and, last but not least, a report on the document 'Unemployment, health and social policy'. In this case, at least, the strategy of information subsidy had been effective.

Some satisfaction was afforded to the UHSG by the reply of the then Minister for Health, Kenneth Clarke to the copy of the 'Leeds Report' he was sent. In a letter dated 18 September, he wrote:

> I did not realise there was any controversy about the connection between unemployment and health. I have always thought that unemployment for any length of time was almost certain to have some adverse effect on peoples' health ... I fear that I do not agree with your economic as opposed to your health research.

The LS research team also seemed rather pleased with what they regarded as a most enthusiastic response by the media to their working paper. This despite the fact that it had been leaked to the press. Had it not been for the UHSG jumping the gun, would they have made a decision to go public with the Working Paper at this stage? One LS researcher felt:

It won't do us any harm. We had a discussion with Alex – Alex phoned us a couple of weeks ago. Then the *Guardian* came down and interviewed us last week … They were told what had been said at the Institute of Statisticians meeting … They were given a couple of papers, and they've based the article on these, in addition to what Alex had done [on 'unemployment-related deaths'] and the UHSG report.

Once the contents of the paper had reached the media in any case, it was felt to be wiser to talk to reporters and make sure they got the facts straight rather than cause more controversy by silence (even after this effort one report managed to demonstrate 'accident proneness' by quoting the LS as containing 500,000 unemployed men rather than 500,000 members in total). In this researcher's opinion: 'Basically the reason the *Guardian* liked it is that there is just enough of a hint … that this is some sort of leak of some "Official Report"'.

They admitted that talking to the press before publication in a journal had brought them in for 'a bit of criticism' and that BBC TV had decided not to cover the story until the 'official report' was published, because it was government data. In fact, only one of the other national daily newspapers carried the story, despite the enthusiasm of the radio stations. This was *The Scotsman*. Other reports of the Working Paper's findings were carried in the *Morning Star* ('Unemployment *is* murder'), *Labour Weekly* ('Research confirms jobless die sooner'), and the Liverpool *Echo* ('Death on the Dole'). A BBC Radio London journalist told me: Once you've got down to death and suicide, what more can you say about it? People only want to hear just so much about things like this'.

This was a fairly common response of media-workers to the issue from this time onwards. One civil servant's view of these events was that:

I knew the balloon was going to go up again … [the LS researchers] sent me a draft of [their] paper some time ago … I don't think that in [their] sample [one] can be as definitive as a lot of people are interpreting it to be. All [they] can do is set out a strong case that there *may* be something. The first draft I saw was somewhat overstated.

Importantly, it seemed to him that: "There is much less hooha about this issue this time round...' However, this official's impression of the LS team's reaction to being the subject of an information subsidy was quite different to their own account. According to one of the research team:

> from what I [the official] could gather, John Fox was by no means pleased about the way it came out in *The Guardian*. I suspect he will write a letter or something [in protest] ... Andrew Veitch [then health correspondent] always takes this sort of line, whenever anything about unemployment and health turns up.

Indeed it was commonly said amongst media-wise researchers that Veitch[3] was not 'typical' of medical journalists and would often give space to less orthodox views when others would ignore them. The civil servant quoted above seems to have been quite correct, also, in predicting that the media and parliamentary 'balloons' would not reach anything like the heights achieved by use of Brenner and Fagin's work in 1981.

The discrepancy between the two accounts of the LS team's reaction is puzzling. On 5 October, a member of the UHSG told me of a conversation that she had had with some people at Social and Community Planning Research, who have close links with City University. The SCPR people had said that OPCS reacted strongly to the 'leak', by reprimanding members of the Working Paper's author group, and 'reminding some of them of their civil service status'. The situation did not seem to justify a great deal of official concern, in view of what was, in comparison to that received by Brenner and Fagin, relatively low media interest. However, at a much later date, some LS researchers looked back with a certain degree of dismay at the aftermath of events in September 1984, feeling that the SSRU had 'had no peace' since then from official suspicion and scrutiny, and that subsequent bids for government money to carry out other studies had been affected.

What may have motivated a certain amount of governmental disquiet over the possible effect of more bad news about the health of the unemployed was the revival of the more social-democratic or 'wet' faction of the Conservative Party in late 1984. This revival had its major opportunity for expression at the annual party conference, which took place 8–12 October. But rumblings were apparent well before this date. On 25 September, a week after the 'leak' of the LS findings, Hugo Young wrote a feature in the *Guardian* entitled 'A valediction on the death of consensus in British politics'. This article touches on many of the themes which were to overtake and incorporate the unemployment and health debate, and describes the movements in opinion which were ironically to make the debate both more relevant to general political discussion and less noteworthy in itself. Young laments several major changes in what he sees as British political traditions. Firstly, the Civil Service: 'Civil servants now find themselves abandoning their customary role of testing the practicality of the politicians' objectives to destruction, and serving up instead the advice they know ministers want to hear'. More generally, Young felt that: "the rules of engagement in public life have been rewritten. In particular, the concepts of neutrality and objectivity, so dear to the civil service mind and so close ... to the very essence of British civilisation, have been abolished'. He warns the Conservatives that if they so profoundly 'politicise British society' as this, formerly quiescent public functionaries, such as bishops, judges and civil servants may be expected to start 'fighting back'.

Echoing the sentiments of the government statisticians involved in and around the debate, a wider range of officials were beginning to formulate the idea of a duty to something beyond 'the government', or as Young puts it, 'the political imperatives of the moment' (Benjamin 1984, Boreham 1984a, 1985, Orchard 1985, Hoinville and Smith 1982; Moser 1980). Early in October, the Archbishop of Canterbury raised the temperature of 'social issues' by giving an outspoken interview to *The Times*, in which he criticised the government's handling of the miners' strike as well as its general economic policies. According to *The Times*: [the Archbishop] denounced unprecedented levels of unemployment, despair and poverty in the community, inequitable sacrifices and those who "treat people as scum"'.

The Conservative Party Conference provided an opportunity for a resurgence of these more liberal ideas, and for the party leadership to be seen to be responding. Shortly before the Conference, Mr David Young, former chairperson of the Manpower Services Commission was appointed as 'the Cabinet's own job creation expert' (according to *The Times* 8 October), to be a Minister without Portfolio and head of a Special Enterprise Unit 'designed to promote job opportunities'.

Notes

1. The numbers in the Government Statistical Service had been reduced from 263 in May 1979 to 193 in March 1984, see Boreham (1984b).
2. The preservation of funding for the social sciences by way of increasing the emphasis symbolically laid upon economics would constitute a topic for a separate research project in the sociology of knowledge, see Flather (1987) which cannot be attempted here. However, the occurrence of this symbolic change is consistent with the argument of the present study.
3. In 1980, Science Editor for Channel Four television.

6

COMPROMISES BETWEEN EXPERTS

The miners' strike, revolt stirring amongst civil servants, protest from the Church of England and disquiet on the government's own left wing shaped the political context in which most of the leading academic protagonists of the debate on unemployment and physical health came together on 26 October, 1984. The occasion was an ESRC-supported workshop on 'Employment and unemployment' held at the Department of Employment (DE). Two papers were scheduled, one by Fox on 'Unemployment and mortality from the OPCS Longitudinal Study', the other by Platt on 'Parasuicide and unemployment in Edinburgh 1968–82'. The organisers were Adrian Sinfield (who was then Professor of Social Policy at Edinburgh University), Michael Hill of the University of Bristol's School of Advanced Urban Studies, and Chris Trinder of the National Institute for Economic and Social Research. Attenders included departmental advisers on economic and social issues from both DHSS and DE.

Fox began his presentation by giving some historical background to the LS work on unemployment, stressing that their early table showing the high mortality of the 'unemployed' (i.e. men 'seeking work' in the week before Census night 1971) had first appeared in a relatively obscure journal in 1979 (Fox 1979), and only been 'picked up' in 1980 by the DHSS CS team. Thus, the controversial table's next appearance, in the *Employment Gazette* of September 1981 (in Ramsden and Smee 1981), had not been the LS team's doing at all. 'The Department of Employment and the DHSS *approached us*,' he related, 'to see if we were interested in doing research on unemployment and health. However, in the end, we went to the MRC and other bodies for our funding' He also pointed out that:

> We did not return to this question of unemployment and health again until the beginning of this year – and that was because I had been invited to a meeting in Australia ... Harvey Brenner was the invited speaker from the USA ... So

I thought, I've got to find some new data, and I started
looking at the unemployment data up to the 1981 Census.

Here Fox reminded his audience of the 'natural history' of Working Paper 18, locating it within the academic cycle of credibility,
rather than the political debate. His introduction was totally
different to that given by David Jones in his presentation of a very
similar paper, based on the same data, to the Institute of Statisticians
conference. This was in accordance with both the very different
audiences, and with the fact that circumstances were now more
highly charged since the 17 September information subsidy.

In looking for his new data in the next five years' follow-up of
the LS sample, it had been found that the overall figure for mortality amongst the unemployed was surprisingly high. In characteristic 'LS style', Fox went on to enumerate, first of all the weaknesses of the study (small numbers of deaths amongst the unemployed, weak and cross-sectional measure of unemployment,
only 1971 data on unemployment available). This was followed
by its strengths: that it is not 'ecological' (that is, it deals with
individuals and not the aggregate groups in Brenner's work), it
includes data on others in the index individual's household, it is
prospective. The rest of his talk was broadly similar to that given
by David Jones in July. At the end, he made an appeal to the
audience for ideas for future work which they would like to see.

The discussion which followed will be reported in some detail
because it represents a rare direct, public confrontation between
the two 'sides' of the debate, uninhibited by the conventions of
academic publishing or a more formal conference setting. There
seemed to be something of a 'comprehension gap' between the LS
team and its audience, which may be common to other confronta-
tions between researchers and policy-makers. The most heated
part of the discussion was on the question of 'health selection',
and here difficulties of comprehension and disagreements of
substance were more or less indissoluble. One Department of
Employment economist was speaking for many participants
when he described 'selection' as 'the crucial issue'. He went on:

Listening to the example you [Fox] gave, perhaps it is my
fault, but I didn't understand it ... much of the excess death
is from smoking-related diseases – and smokers are more
likely to be unreliable workers as well as more likely to get
lung cancer. How have you dealt with this sort of problem?

In his reply, Fox made what was probably his first publicly contested attempt to explain the significance of the 'wearing off of selection', as applied to the problem of the effect of unemployment on health:

If you have a group of people with, shall we call it, a natural mortality level – let's just assume for a moment that there is no social mobility. Then if, by your sample selection, you oversample people who are unhealthy at the start of follow-up, then mortality from this group should be high to begin with, but you'd expect it to go down [as the very sick members of the group 'die off', and the less sick recover]. On the other hand, if you take a group where you've selected *out* the sick people, you'd expect *their* initial mortality to be *low* [in relation to that of the whole population which contains both sick and healthy], and then to rise back towards the natural [population] level.

This is what was found when looking at the unemployed men in the LS. Fox supplemented this explanation by some comments directly referring to his earlier work on the 'healthy worker effect'. In his previous work on industrial diseases, low mortality had been found for all groups of workers at the beginning of cohort studies, which rises back to the 'natural level' over time. This approach had been used in studies of asbestos and other industrial hazards. As a result, studies of industrial hazards now no longer compare the mortality of workers with possibly hazardous substances with that of the population as a whole, but only with groups of other workers, who may be expected to be similarly 'selected for good health' by the recruitment process. The idea that 'health selection wears off' is therefore a well established one, though in other fields of inquiry.

In the LS, if I take people by economic position and look at trends in health, there is [amongst the unemployed] a *rise* in the level of mortality over time [similar to that found in 'healthy workers'. If you take the sick group, it goes in quite the opposite direction. The 'seeking work' group is artificially biased the other way from what you are suggesting [i.e. only the relatively healthy *are* seeking work as opposed to defining themselves as permanently sick] ... I'm not claiming this is conclusive. But the interpretation at this time is that our group is positively, not negatively, selected for health.

The same line of argument was than taken up by another government economist:

What if there was some variable, not measured in the LS, which caused *both* unemployment *and*, say, suicidal tendencies? then you will generate the kind of association you have found, even though it is not a causal relationship. We know that assortative mating is strong. Now, although I think the high mortality of the wives is one of the strongest aspects of your data, we cannot ignore the possibility that emotionally disturbed people, say, may marry each other.

Fox replied to this that there was no correlation found between the death rates, or ages of death, of spouses in the LS . His antagonist persisted: 'We all know there is assortative mating by class, education, culture, etcetera. I don't know if that would be expected to lead to similar levels of mortality'. But Fox was not to be moved:

If these people had some reason for higher mortality, then eventually they would have to die out, and thus their contribution to the group's mortality rate would wear off over time. In the long term, the mortality rate of any group some of whose members were 'selected for poor health' would, therefore *have* to fall. If I've initially put in more of such people, some of them should die off in the first year, so next year there should be a smaller proportion of them in the whole group, and the next year even smaller, and so on …

Another economic adviser asked: 'But what if the characteristic is one which isn't like illness, but some trait which is likely to trigger mortality at more widely distributed times?' In response, Fox argued that there was no 'medical model' of illness in use which could make sense of such a pattern of deaths widely and randomly spaced in time, which were nevertheless 'triggered' by the same sort of underlying 'characteristic' that could be used to explain unemployment. Eventually, one of the economic advisers became more specific about what the 'unmeasured factor' which could trigger mortality might be:

We only have fragmentary evidence on this, but what there is tends to suggest that people who are unemployed smoke and drink more heavily on average than the people in employment, but this is while they are *employed*. When they are actually unemployed, they smoke and drink less. Now, this is precisely the kind of factor that will predispose people to unemployment and also kill them off earlier.

But Fox returned to the fact that the high death rate of the unemployed in the early period of follow up did not 'wear off', which would be expected if a significant number of those found to be seeking work at one point in tine were being killed off by something which predated their uneaployment, no matter what this was. Even if a group had high mortality because it contained a lot of smokers, for example, eventually the smokers would all have died and the death rate in the group would have to fall.

Here I must make it clear that, in common with most members of the UHSG, as well as a wide range of other participants in the debate, I did not fully understand this argument in late 1984. The phrases in square brackets within the quotations from my field notes of Fox's talk have been added at the time of writing in order to make comprehension easier for the reader. Understanding the 'wearing off of selection' argument was something which happened to a relatively small group almost in the manner of a 'conversion experience' or paradigm-switch (in my case, during the autumn of 1986). What happened next in this workshop also seemed at the time to resemble a conversion experience on the part of one of the economists. But it did not take place on the basis of the arguments about the wearing off of selection. Rather, it was a product of the perceived strength of the argument that spouses of the unemployed were (despite 'assortative mating') *not* very likely to be similarly 'selected' for poor health. It was also based on the perception that the work embodied in the second paper (Steve Platt's) was amenable to a different kind of research programme which might appropriately shift the focus of the academic debate from economic policy to policies of alleviating the effects of unemployment.

After the tea-break, during which the participants tended to break up into 'camps', statisticians on one side and economists and government researchers on the other, Platt spoke on the findings which he and Norman Kreitman had just had published in the *BMJ*, four days previously (Platt and Kreitman 1984, see also Platt and Kreitman 1985, Platt 1986a). As was stated in their second draft of this paper, submitted in August, Platt now repeated that these were 'preliminary results' and that a fuller version would be published in another journal, *Psychological Medicine* in the following year. He summed up his talk:

> I must make it quite clear that we tend to conclude – how can I put this now? – that our findings are not incompatible with a causal role for unemployment. That is the most

conservative way of saying it that I can think of. But we point out that we are not putting forward a monocausal theory. We know that lots of these people have alcohol problems and criminal records and that kind of thing. We are aware that there are self-selection factors involved.

After this talk, the second person to ask a question was a prominent member of the 'other side' of the argument, one of the economists. He felt that:

The question is, what ought one to be doing about or in response to this balance of evidence? That's a very big agenda. I think the SAPU people [Prof Peter Warr's research group at the Social and Applied Psychology unit at Sheffield University] find that, for young people, going in a YOP course has as good an effect as being in employment.

The economist continued to enumerate a series of possible 'alleviations': extension of the long-term rate of benefit to the unemployed, Community Programmes, wider availability of part-time work. 'If the "poverty effect" visible in ecological data were significant, then the first measure night be the most important', he suggested. After some more questions and discussion on the combined effects of recession and inflation on people other than those actually unemployed, Platt stepped out of the specialist social-psychologist role, as if to extend an appeal for dialogue to the economists present:

I'd like to say something about inflation – here I'm going to get sat on by an economist – we use unemployment as an indicator of the state of the economy which is reasonably reliable. What worries me is the extent to which it gives one a true picture of the state of the economy at the present time. Whichever indicator you read: inflation, GNP, income per caput, etc., you get a different impression ... Is this very silly?

To which one of the economists replied: 'It is very sensible ... You've hit on something very important. There are clearly times when unemployment is high and real incomes are growing ... Unemployment rates are good indicators of the state of the unemployed, but not for the state of the employed.'

This exchange illustrates the beginnings of a promising 'translation', a member of each group tentatively extending an offer of their respective definitions of the situation as a 'resource' to the other side. The rest of the discussion centred around the psychology of parasuicide and reflected both the interests of a large section of the audience, and of the MRC Unit in which Platt worked. When the meeting ended, some participants 'hung around', forming small groups. I asked the economist who had proposed 'policy changes' (I shall call him 'E') if I had heard him aright? Was he really proposing a change in the agenda, from academic argument to discussion of concrete measures to protect that health of the unemployed? He replied, firmly, that he was. The sort of research now needing to be done was exemplified by Jennie Popay's study of how health visitors and social workers dealt with the problem of having a growing proportion of unemployed in their caseloads. More research was also needed, however, on 'precipitating/mediating effects and how to intervene'. I asked if he thought there would now be a lobby within the DHSS for the extension of the long term rate of benefit to the unemployed. But this, he felt, was crying for the moon, 'It's a question of priorities'. At this point we were joined by a member of the LS team, who was clutching a note passed over to him by 'E' during the discussion of Platt's paper. 'Can we [the LS team] rely on you to say this sort of thing in the Department?' the researcher asked. The economist replied, cautiously, 'I'm convinced. It's just a question of whether I can be *seen* to be convinced.' The researcher urged him, 'It's the sort of thing we need you to say'. (The LS researchers were at this time negotiating with the OPCS for permission to carry on linking post-1981 vital event data to the 1971 sample). 'E' replied that he found the evidence that the wives of unemployed men also had a higher risk of mortality the most persuasive piece of evidence so far, but he went on 'Come on, now, you and I know ... that the DHSS is very hard to move on this sort of thing.' He insisted that 'It would be mistaken to aim this stuff [the findings of the LS and of Platt and Kreitman's study] at the macro-economic debate ... If this governnent wouldn't make a U-turn in 1981, how much less can they afford to now.' Rather, he felt that if research was to continue being seen as a useful adjunct in the debate on social policy relating to the unemployed, it must be removed from the discussion on economic policy, and redirected towards problems of 'intervention' and 'alleviation'. Future proposals for research should therefore, he argued, emphasise two features: improved estimates of the costs of labour market policies, including costs at the 'macro' level (for example, to the Health Service), and recommendations on how to carry out limited interventions directed at vulnerable groups. Potentially, Platt's work was more amenable to this kind of change in emphasis than that of Fox and colleagues. An emphasis on individual vulnerability and intervention was also in general accord with a strong strand in the research programme of the MRC Unit for Epidemiological Studies in Psychiatry.

The findings reported in Fox's talk were published on 8 December in *The Lancet* (Moser *et al.* 1981). But by this time, there was not a great deal more to be said about the 1971–81 follow-up of the LS's 'unemployed' men and their wives. The material in the published paper was essentially the same as in the working paper reported in the media the previous September. In the discussion of 'selection', the published paper is rather more explicit than the working paper or David Jones' rendering of it. The 'wearing off' to be expected in a group selected for poor health is, in *The Lancet* version, spelt out as due to 'the high initial mortality of those selected on the basis of ill-health [which would mean that] the proportion of sick men in this category would decline over time … as has been observed in other areas of our work '.

Both in *The Lancet* paper and the working paper, a far more cautious attitude is taken towards extrapolation of the findings to the unemployed of the 1980s, than that exhibited in the 'leaked' *Guardian* report of September 1984. As unemployment has become a 'more common experience', has its severity decreased, due to a reduction of stigma? On the other hand, average duration of unemployment has increased. *The Lancet* paper promises that further analysis of the LS cohort will answer this question in due time.

There was little media response. The UHSG produced a deliberately co-ordinated onslaught on the letters page of *The Lancet*, with letters coming from Steve Watkins, Silvia Tilford (a member of the Leeds Report drafting group), Gill Westcott, and Scott-Samuel. The latter included in some detail (including two tables) the extrapolation of Moser *et al.*'s findings to the 1980s unemployed population. Even taking the lowest and most conservative estimate, Scott-Samuel claimed, there had been an annual excess of deaths 'due to unemployment' of 1,034 (combining unemployed men and their wives). 'For every 1,000 men seeking work, 1.94 men and 0.98 wives will die each year as a result of unemployment' he concluded, offering a 'Brenneresque' ready-reckoning method for any local planning department, or indeed, pressure group, to use.

Research to policy: in the balance

It would seen that those who had for long suspected, and sought to demonstrate, that unemployment damaged physical health, and wished to persuade policy-makers of this were now taking the offensive. What seemed to have taken place at the seminar reported above was another turning point, where the weight of evidence had finally swayed at least one civil service professional. However, what followed matches more closely the fourth phase of Manning and Downs' model, which has been characterised by Downs as a 'twilight zone' of declining interest. This did not happen because of any scientific work 'successfully' questioning the knowledge claims of the British Regional Heart Study, the LS or the Edinburgh MRC Unit, but rather as part of the increasing tendency of this work to be interpreted differently according to the uses made of it by different groups, and not to be directly challenged.

On 14 November 1984, the UHSG meeting noted with satisfaction that Kenneth Clarke, both in his letter to the director of the Nuffield Centre for Health Services Studies who had published the UHSG's 'Leeds Report', and in a speech to the MIND annual conference, had admitted that unemployment was damaging to health. But, the minutes note, 'the change in governnent attitude had not resulted in any policy change'.

The Labour Party now took up the question, independently of the UHSG. Michael Meacher asked a string of Parliamentary Questions between October 1984 (shortly after the 'leak' of the LS results) June 1985 about both the LS research and the policy proposals in the 'Leeds Report'. Rather dramatically, Labour Front Bench health spokesperson Frank Dobson is quoted (in *Labour Weekly*, 4 January) as saying: 'At first the Government pretended that there was no link between unenployment and ill-health and deaths. Recently they have had to begin owning up to those links ... That means that now, through their policies, they are knowingly killing people'.

On 10 January, *New Scientist* devoted a full page to a feature entitled 'Death on the dole', reporting that the LS results' will be taken up by Opposition MPs in the coming weeks as further evidence of the inhumanity of the government's economic policies'. As one night expect, the 'wearing off' argument makes its first 'popular' media appearance here, in a popular-scientific journal. Unfortunately, it is not phrased in a way which seems well calculated to clarify the idea, even to the scientifically-trained uninitiated.

At the UHSG's first meeting of 1985, on 16 January, it was felt that:

> we were not 'over the top' yet as regards government attitudes, research findings, and the Unemployment Health and Social Policy report [the 'Leeds Report']. The acknowledgement by Kenneth Clarke of the health-damaging effects of unemployment needed to be translated into action; the steadily more conclusive findings of research needed wider dissemination.

Other participants gave far more importance to Clarke's statement. One felt that it was a 'key event', signalling a major departure fron the position of other Ministers (particularly Gerard Vaughan). This meant that civil servants no longer felt they had to defend what some now saw as a 'virtually indefensible position', and could turn their attention with some relief to designing policies to alleviate the effects of unemployment on health. According to this view, Clarke had also helped to spike the guns of the UHSG and their sympathisers by placing the issue outside of epidemiology and firmly into the sphere of economic policy.

A needle and a haystack

Against this backqround of debate, the last face-to-face confrontation between members of the 'core group' took place on 1 February 1985. This took place at a workshop in London, organised by the Centre for Economic Policy Research, an independent policy research organisation. Both speakers and audience were invited. The workshop was partly financed by the DHSS, and was seen by some as an opportunity for civil servants to debate with members of the UHSG without taking a fixed position on the possibility that unemployment could be harmful, due to the statement made by Kenneth Clarke the previous September. Had he not done so, one remarked, such a debate would not have been possible.

An eminent group of speakers had been invited from various parts of Europe, their expenses paid by the DHSS, as part of its ongoing support for the Centre's programme of research on 'human resources'. The organiser of the workshop was Prof Roderick Floud of Birkbeck College, an economic historian, who also chaired. It took place in a cheerful and lively atmosphere. By now, most of the researchers in the 'core group' knew both each other and the representatives of 'Manifesto' Community Medicine who had been most involved, Watkins and Scott-Samuel. It was a welcome opportunity for widely dispersed members of the network to meet. A considerable number of notes were passed back and forth during the more formal sessions, and breaks were busily occupied, both by friendly chat and by what was described as 'horse-trading' (that is, discussion of possible government funding for research) between academics and civil servants (three were present from DHSS and one from the Department of Employment).

The first paper to be presented was Derek Cook's, another version of the Institute of Statisticians' paper. Once again, he made heavy use of the dietary study of Doyle and Crawford, somewhat strangely in view of the fact that this study does not specify whether any of the breadwinners of the Hackney or Hampstead samples were actually unemployed. On this occasion, he also criticised the suggestion in Gravelle, Hutchinson and Stern's 1981 paper that a 'robust effect' could be isolated in time-series work by 'better statistical techniques'. Cook felt this was a 'pious hope', and that 'superior statistical technique will not be the answer'.

Cook's discussant was Jon Stern, who felt it had been a 'very good exposition of the problems as I see them'. He agreed that more time-series analysis was pointless, despite what had been said in the paper of which he was co-author ('I didn't write that sentence') and felt that: 'The fundamental methodological problem is what is known as selection bias'.

It was not just a question of whether unemployed people were physiologically 'diseased'. The meaning of 'selection' shifts according to the argument in which it is used, and the people who use it. Stern's usage, for example, was based on the idea that there is a normal distribution of 'human capital' factors such as intelligence in any population, and that those who found themselves unemployed might be drawn from the 'lower' end of this distribution. He now argued that 'we do now have three large scale good studies. It would be stupid to deny that there is some effect of unemployment on physical health and mortality. The effect is probably small rather than large ... But we have found the needle in the haystack' Policy advisers had, it seems, adopted the published British research as the basis for what now seemed to be an emerging consensus. Stern went on to ask where 'we should go from here'. He was in favour of 'small scale studies' and 'action research' to investigate 'mediating effects', that is, the pathways by which the now admitted *'ceteris paribus* effect' of unemployment on health operated.

One of the officials present then took up a theme of the discussion following the October ESRC workshop:

> What do we mean by 'policy'? As a DHSS official, policy in this area means affecting the kind of policy variables that are under the control of the DHSS. One problem is that the health effects have been used as a weapon in the war about macro-economic policy. Fine, terrific. But those kinds of policies are under the control of the Prime Minister and the Chancellor of the Exchequer.

Further interesting information and discussion was forthcoming from papers that followed, much of which has been written up elsewhere (*CEPR Bulletin* March 1985; Whiteside 1987, 1988). But from the point of view of the present account, the other important discussion took place between Platt and Hugh Gravelle, who had been invited by Floud to be discussant to Platt's paper.

This discussion was scheduled as the first after tea. Gravelle, it will be remembered had been an author of the influential paper co-authored with Stern and Gillian Hutchinson, criticising Brenner's work in 1981. During the break Gravelle foreswore the social mixing, took his tea back into the seminar room, and proceeded to write a series of equations on the blackboard. Platt's paper once again presented the Edinburgh Regional Poisoning Treatment Centre study, which included both 'ecological' correlations between unemployment and parasuicide rates in different areas of Lothian Region, and time-series data on the rate of parasuicide in unemployed individuals (see Platt and Kreiban 1985). Offering a 'translation' of the work as a resource to the range of workshop participants, Platt began by remarking: 'The origin of the project was in the growing interest in unemployment and health and the thought that I could exploit a unique data set'.

The main points of the paper that are relevant for the discussion which then took place were as follows:

- Unemployment and parasuicide were highly correlated over time, at least until 1983.
- Unemployment rose, the proportion of parasuicide cases who were unemployed also rose

- Over time, the relative risk of parasuicide amongst the unemployed (compared to that among the employed) began at a very high level, then fell, and then stabilised at around eleven to one.
- Cross-sectional data showed that areas of high unenployment tended to be areas with high rates of parasuicide, but this correlation was reduced to statistical insignificance when a measure of poverty was introduced as a control variable.

In reply, Gravelle emphasised the economists' distinctive approach: 'you have to start with basic models. Firstly a production function – an aetiological model that summarizes your hypotheses about the relationship between unemployment rates and parasuicide rates ... Secondly, you need a model of behaviour'.

He went on to give the fullest and most explicit account to date of the economists' approach' to the problem of the relationship between unemployment and health. Gravelle's first two criticisms of Platt's paper were purely technical. He pointed out that the proportion of parasuicides who are unemployed is bound to increase as the unemployment rate rises (just as the proportion of, say, red-headed people who are unemployed would increase as the rate of unemployment rises). Therefore the amount of parasuicide in the population as a whole which can be attributed to unemployment (the 'attributable risk') must rise as unemployment rises. Next, as in his critique of Brenner, Gravelle proposed that if Platt and Kreitman's time-series was broken into two, the correlations would disappear for each separate period. Turning to the 'ecological' data, Gravelle picked up the point that when poverty was controlled, the cross-sectional correlation between unemployment rates and parasuicide rates in Edinburgh enumeration districts disappeared. That suggested to him 'severe problems of multicollinearity. That means that all the results which do not include poverty as a measure must be biased'.

There was an anomaly, he thought, between the time-series and the cross-sectional data: namely that across areas with different rates of unemployment, parasuicide rates rose steadily with unemployment: the higher the unemployment rates, the higher the parasuicide rate. But across *time periods* with different rates of unemployment, the *relative* risk of parasuicide behaved less consistently. As the unemployment rate rose, the relative risk of parasuicide in unemployed men first fell, and then stabilised. He proposed that this anomaly in fact offered the key to explaining the 'true' link between unemployment and parasuicide. The data could now be interpreted as showing that at the beginning of the period of the Edinburgh study, the high rates of parasuicide amongst the unemployed were entirely due to 'personal characteristics' (as Platt himself had argued in 1982). The finding that parasuicide was highest amongst higher social class individuals who were unemployed could also be explained in this way – they were the ones with the most 'personal problems' (i.e. they were unemployed despite a relatively favourable labour market position). People with 'personal problems' were also concentrated in poor areas, hence the high rates of self-destructive behaviour in these areas. However, Gravelle admitted that there were two factors operating to produce rates of unemployment: as well as 'personal characteristics', the demand for labour also plays a part. As unemployment rose, the second of the two possible determinants of the 'propensity to unemployment' (i.e. the demand for labour) took over from the first ('personal characteristics'), hence one would expect the 'new' unemployed to have better mental health and a lower rate of parasuicide, which is what the data show. This point had also been admitted by Moser and her LS co-workers when they asked whether the mortality rates of men unenployed at the 1981 Census could be expected to be as elevated as that of men unemployed in 1971.

This was an impressive presentation, the effect of which was heightened by the presence of complicated-looking equations on the blackboard. The intensity of the confrontation between Platt and Gravelle meant that the closing discussion of 'policy', introduced by Jennie Popay, was conducted in a somewhat muted atmosphere. Frustrated at an apparent return to the 'loop' of technical debate, she protested that: 'You're asking for more research in this area than ever gets asked for to justify policy change in other areas. The only similar case I can think of is with inequalities in health. You ask for so much rigour, that you end up with rigor mortis'.

Floud then turned to 'our colleagues from the DHSS', and asked their opinions. One research administrator felt, like Stern, that: 'The approaches we can adopt have to relate to services. Some measures to help improve the level of living of people who are unemployed is the direction we'd prefer'. In contrast to this an administrator thought: 'There are some policy implications we

can take on board and some we cannot. The implications of raising benefit, if that was what the research implied, are such that the
present government would be unlikely to envisage, let's face it'.
Gravelle himself was more cautious about 'intervention'. If his
interpretation of the Edinburgh figures were correct, then unemployment, poverty, area of residence and suicidal behaviour
could still all be due to personal characteristics. 'Unless you have
got some model, just going in and intervening might not tell you
much,' he warned.

The evening after the meeting, considerable disquiet was expressed by some participants at the outcome of the day's proceedings. As one put it: 'I don't think what Hugh did was on. Steve has
always played it straight, always played the game according to
the rules. If Hugh was going to attack him like that, at least he
should have warned him'. Plans were made to liaise with Platt
over 'how to get round' the 'problem' pointed out by Gravelle.
One statistician's opinion was that Gravelle's presentation had
been 'rubbish', implying that it was not really worth bothering
about. Between this day and the end of my period of observation
of the debate, Gravelle's rebuttal of Platt and Kreitman's work
was never published in a refereed journal, and Platt was therefore
under no obligation (according to 'the rules') to reply to it. He sent
a copy of the equations to Derek Cook, who found the notation
confusing, and both researchers were too busy to devote the
necessary time to clarification. The links proposed that evening
between Platt, Stern and Cook (sociologist, economist and statistician) were never re-activated.

Stalemate

An account of the CEPR workshop was written up and published
in the next edition of the *CEPR Bulletin* in March. Several members of the workshop were dismayed at having been given no
chance to see it beforehand. It came into the hands of the UHSG in
a roundabout way. A copy was sent to Michael Meacher in his
capacity as Shadow Secretary of State for Health and Social Security, and his research assistant forwarded it to Scott-Samuel,
whom she knew as a member of the Labour Party's Front Bench
advisory group with this special interest. The comment on Platt's
paper was that 'his methodology was heavily criticised in the
discussion which followed [his paper]. Without further research,
these conclusions will not gain widespread acceptance.' The report

of the workshop concluded: 'It is necessary to ascertain what aspects of health are affected by unemployment and what remedial measures can be taken to protect the health of unemployed people'.

If one were to agree fully with Gravelle, the implication could have been that it was unlikely any aspects of health were greatly affected by unemployment, and remedial measures in the form of labour market policies would be wasted. A more logical response might have been to extend more 'help' to 'vulnerable people' in general, but their employment status would therefore be incidental. More complex interpretations of research were only partially assimilated, even those which pointed away from any implication of unemployment in damaging health, when they ran counter to, or were irrelevant to, notions about alleviation. Jon Stern felt that Gravelle himself had imposed too high a requirement for 'rigour' for purposes of policy-related debate. 'What is a gospel of academic purity and is not the way the world works,' he remarked later. A more appropriate response would be

> *not* to wait until research has come up with 'the answer'; rather it is to be modest in policy design and, particularly, to build up policies so that they can be developed or discarded as experience shows up their relevance to the problem and to the strengths and weaknesses of the initial policy design.

In some ways the outcome of the workshop, at least in the *CEPR Bulletin*'s account (see also Gravelle 1985), was a striking reversal of that of the ESRC workshop of October 1984. One of the major pieces of research in the debate was now redefined as something which 'would not gain widespread acceptance'. However, contrary to this conclusion, Steve Platt continued to be invited to address important academic and professional meetings (such as the Royal College of Psychiatrists' annual conference in July 1985) throughout the rest of my period of observing the debate, and he was also invited to write an editorial on the topic for the *British Journal of Psychiatry*, which appeared in the late summer of 1986 (Platt 1986b). The notion that unemployment increased the risk of suicidal behaviour continued to be widely accepted in subsequent literature as one of the firmest findings of the entire corpus of research on unemploynent and health. In Jon Stern's opinion, this acceptance was justified because Gravelle's critique while methodologically correct had not necessarily damaged the substance of the argument. A more rigorous specification of Platt's model could have withstood criticism more effectively. As Platt colourfully described it shortly afterwards, a goal had been scored, but it was hard to know which team had scored it.

It was in some ways rather strange to see time (from February 1985 to 1987) pass without any further testing of the ideas which had been so hotly debated between 1981 and 1984. After the CEPR workshop there were no further meetings of the 'core group' and no further debate between core group members in academic journals. Could the Edinburgh data on parasuicide have been used in such a way as to 'get round' Gravelle's objections? The question was never answered.

What appeared a promising line of further enquiry at the beginning of 1985 was to be found in the British Regional Heart Study. The team at the Royal Free had interviewed nearly 8,000 men between 1978 and 1980 in twenty-four towns in England, Scotland and Wales, towns chosen to give representation of regions with different rates of heart disease (for further explanation of the setting up of the Heart Study, see Chapter 10). In 1982 they had successfully applied for some additional funding to mail out follow-up questionnaires to all subjects (men age 40–64 when they were first interviewed) asking about, amongst other things, their experience of unemployment. Over 95 per cent of the men returned their questionnaires. As a result, the study had by 1985 assembled a set of data including the men's jobs and state of health (including such 'objective' measures as blood pressure, ECG, blood fats and lung function tests) before the onset of the economic crisis. Unemployment rates in some towns had quadrupled, others had been relatively unaffected. A team member pointed out that it was a 'natural experiment' of a type not often possible, which had fallen into their laps. In the longer term, any relationship between employment histories and mortality could be estimated net of the possible effect of ill health.

However in the autumn of 1984, while the unemployment follow-up data was still being collected, the Regional Heart Study application for a further five-year programme grant from the MRC (its third) was unsuccessful. As a consequence, Derek Cook had to abandon his work for a PhD using the follow-up data on unemployment and mortality experience of the 7,735 men. To embark on a PhD when it was not certain that all the data could be collected was too risky. His new topic was to be an investigation of lung function in relation to social class, town of residence, and smoking. Cook's decision to re-direct his efforts was taken quite abruptly. *The Lancet* of 8 December 1984 had published an optmistic letter in which he spelt out the promise of the study in relation to the question of the relationship between unemployment and health:

> The suggestion arising from this study is that those men who have early evidence of disease may become unemployed more readily and remain unemployed for longer than men who are healthy. This possibility cannot be confirmed from the preliminary cross-sectional analysis, a more dynamic view of the unemployment/health relationship is needed.

Obtaining this 'dynamic view' was the purpose of the postal questionnaire, sent out five years after each man had first been interviewed, and therefore staggered over the years 1983 to 1985. In conjunction with the measurements made at initial examination it was hoped to:

> examine the extent to which men have been selectively forced out or kept out of the workforce because of ill-health ... The Regional Heart Study should be able to provide detailed information on the dynamics of the unemployment and health interrelationship and to quantify this 'selection of the fittest'.

In the event, the Regional Heart Study did receive generous funding from other bodies, such as the British Heart Foundation. However, the need to change the emphasis of the work and to be more willing to prepare papers for publicly visible occasions (to attract yet further funding) produced a new set of priorities for Cook. He firmly believed, by late 1986, that smoking amongst the unemployed could be shown to account for both a raised risk of unemployment and for the 'randomly triggered' higher mortality, spaced out over time, found amongst those men in the LS who had been unemployed at the time of the 1971 Census. The spacing of the 'excess deaths', he felt, could be explained by the fact that people had taken up smoking at different ages, and so reached the end of the 'latency period' for lung cancer (the cause of death most in excess of average amongst the middle aged and older 'unemployed' men in the LS) at different times. As the British Regional Heart Study had data on the age at when men took up smoking, state of health at the beginning of the study (and the recession), employment history, and mortality, the claims in *The Lancet* letter did not seem exaggerated. This work was not done, however, at least not in the subsequent five years.

In 1991, Derek Cook took up a post as senior lecturer at St George's Hospital Medical School By this time, he had a PhD student, Joan Morris, working on the full set of data on the employment histories of the Heart Study men. Her work concentrated on ways in which unemployment affected the amount the men consulted their GPs. Cook and Morris had also considered pursuing the relationship between employment histories and previous health, thereby directly testing some of the hypotheses about 'personal characteristics' and health prior to unemployment. However, there were problems concerning the 'ownership' of the data, which remained at the Royal Free. Because of this, and because, unlike the Economic and Social Research Council (ESRC), the MRC does not oblige data to be made publicly available through the UK Data Archive, it seemed unlikely that any further progress would be made.

7

A TWILIGHT ZONE

Unemployment and health in general practice

One new study of unemployment's effect on health did appear in 1985. This was the 'Calne study', a longitudinal case-control study in which the cases were all patients of a single general practice. It was highly relevant to the original interests of DHSS civil servants who became involved in the debate because it claimed to show increases in demand for health care associated with factory closures.

In 1982, Harris Meats, the major employer in the country town of Calne, Wiltshire, made their entire workforce redundant. The first reported findings of the study were that redundant workers and their spouses were significantly more likely to consult the GP, but not *after* being dismissed. The rise in consultations took place during the extended 'anticipation' period during which workers were aware that the factory was likely to be closed. Redundant patients were, furthermore, more likely than controls to be seen as sufficiently ill to warrant referral to hospital out-patients departments for specialist advice. In March of 1986, a fascinating account written by Beale about the process by which this research came to be done, was published in the *BMJ* (Beale 1986). The 'idea' of using the information from his general practice's register of patients to investigate the impact of the closure is depicted as 'abruptly' occurring to him in the spring of 1983 while he was 'giving the lawn its first haircut'.

Like several other researchers (such as Fox) in their 'public' discovery accounts, Beale distanced himself from any possible 'political' motives. However, he was aware that the imminent closure of the major employer in his area might 'be affecting our practice workload.' This accomplishment of motive is followed by a gesture towards 'science':

> In Cambridge I had been allowed the ultimate privilege of a British science education. The master of my college had won a Nobel prize for work on DNA ... I remembered with

> pleasure the research project I had done for a year after
> Second MB; I had learned to ... define aims, to shuffle index
> cards, to tabulate results ... I was familiar with the infra-
> structure of science at least.

His account of his own 'Pilgrims progress' through the project
is disarmingly honest about mistakes, confusion and the temptation to draw conclusions from incomplete data. Yet it does
portray the process as cumulative, as a progress through error
towards the discovery of truth 'out there'. Beale described his
mood in various emotional terms: 'I was hooked ... Creativity is
close to madness it is said. I could not have survived the next year
without a demonic mania that had developed. I now had an
obsession'. After the tedious work of looking through company
files and medical records to identify his cases and controls, and
trace their medical histories: 'I began to be naughty. I craved for
results and repeatedly compiled data from incomplete samples'.

To his horror, even the completed work showed no change in
illness following redundancy: 'months of work and nothing to
show for it'. However, the fact that the practice's own cleaner had
previously been made redundant during an earlier rationalisation
at Harris Meats caused a 'flash of insight':

> I suddenly understood the importance of something I had
> known for four years: there had been ... earlier redundan-
> cies from the factory ... Did morbidity change with the
> threat of job loss two years before the factory closure? Yes, it
> did. But could I prove it?

At this point, by chance, he met, socially, a medical statistician
who was looking for part-time work (Susan Nethercott) and
'With enormous relief, I handed her the numbers to crunch'. Next,
Beale discovered the Joint Working Party on Unemployment and
Health of the Royal College of General Practitioners and sought
advice from Ian Russell, their statistical adviser. Russell queried
the statistical technique that had been used. Now, using some
money from the Science Foundation Board of the Royal College of
GPs, Nethercott set about re-aggregating the data. This took up
the month of October 1984. The paper was eventually successfully
submitted to the *Journal of the Royal College of General Practitioners*.

The first journalist to pick the study up was Andrew Veitch of
the *Guardian*, who had also been the only one to write about the
Regional Heart Study in 1982. Like Cook and his colleagues, Beale
had made no effort to 'subsidy' his work, and Veitch commented

that full-time medical correspondents (in distinction to the experience of Dinwoodie and Christie of *The Scotsman*) on papers which could afford such things, did regularly scan journals, although the *Journal of the Royal College of General Practitioners* was one which he only looked at when he had 'nothing else to read'. Unlike the Regional Heart Study, however, and perhaps because the memory of the papers by Smee and Ramsden and Gravelle *et al.* had faded by late 1985, the Calne study's impact expanded from coverage in the *Guardian*. Beale described the media response and his own reaction to it: 'countless interviews', his home full of film technicians, the telephone ringing incessantly. The culmination of all this was a summons from the BBC itself, and then yet more findings: 'After the weekend, "Auntie" came, but, more important, Susan had found more significant results, the hub of another paper. To the addict, the fix is everything'.

The next paper from the Calne study to receive media attention was published on 22 December 1986 (Beale and Nethercott 1986d). It resulted once again in requests to appear on radio and TV. Andrew Veitch's fairly small piece in the *Guardian* was headlined 'Redundancy "affects health for years"'. The new finding was that workers most affected by the period of 'anticipation' were those with previous experience of unemployment. Those with previously stable work histories, however, suffered more after redundancy. Veitch still feels that, even so 'ministers have been reluctant to accept that the stress of unemployment has had a significant effect on the nation's health'.

There was, however, no 'official response' to Beale's research. A critique of its methods appeared amongst academic epidemiologists. But this seems to have arisen as part of the competition for research territory: epidemiologists were not particuarly pleased that such a widely acknowledged study had been carried out by a general practitioner. The critique does not appear to have entered into policy debate.

Occupationless health

As if to sum up the debate from the mid-1970s to 1985, a series of articles by Richard Smith entitled 'Occupationless health' appeared in the *BMJ* between late October of 1985 and February of 1986. It is difficult to classify the series as part of the 'academic' or 'public' debates on unemployment and health. This difficulty is not accidental, but reflects the way in which the public debate was increasingly conducted without reference to the academic one.

Writing 'Occupationless health' was a considerable task for a non-specialist who was at the same time one of the *BMJ*'s assistant editors (in mid-1990 Smith was to become editor of the journal). It may be viewed as something which Smith did as part of the 'cycle of credibility' followed by serious medical journalists. He had previously written series on alcohol and prison medicine, and followed 'Occupationless health' with one on research funding. The title of the series implies a 'public' aim, and in content the articles were in the form of a series of reviews of both research and policy responses. The view of the UHSG was that having such a comprehensive review readily available, and the fact that it had appeared in such a 'respectable' journal would add solidity to their case in policy debate.[1]

Richard Smith was an Edinburgh graduate who had completed his 'house jobs' and then worked and travelled in the Far East for some time. On returning to Britain, he had not gone back into clinical medicine but 'fallen on his feet' into an assistant editorial post at the *BMJ*, which he made his career. He felt strongly on the question of unemployment, and, like other sympathetic journalists such as Bryan Christie and Robbie Dinwoodie, was disappointed at the lack of response his work. The content of the articles will not be dealt with in detail here, as the research has been discussed in other chapters.

While planning the series, Smith approached a small group including Scott-Samuel, Platt and Cook with a request that they read over some or all of the articles before publication to 'check factual details'. The group he chose as his 'experts' might, therefore, be regarded as somewhat weighted towards the 'Manifesto' end of the spectrum, but in the first paper, 'Bitterness, shame, emptiness, waste: an introduction to unemployment and health', he states: 'the evidence linking unemployment with poor psychological health , is much stronger than that linking it with poor physical health'. and: 'Studies on how unemployment affects physical health cannot match the sophistication of the psychological studies'.

What was new in this paper was Smith's summing-up not of the outcome of research, but of the way research had been conducted:

> Sadly, although unemployment began to increase dramatically in Britain more than five years ago, no study was ever

set up to study specifically the effects of unemployment on mortality or indeed any other measure of health. Instead, clever use had to be made of data from studies set up for other purposes ... Some people to whom I spoke thought that the government had deliberately discouraged research on unemployment and health, because it did not want any data produced that might make continuing with present economic policies more difficult.

Smith had 'heard of at least two ... cases from England where applications ... had been rejected more on political than scientific grounds.' But, he goes on 'others I spoke to subscribed less to this conspiracy theory and more to the idea that doctors' leaders had been slow to wake up to the importance of unemployment to health' (Smith 1985). He also mentions the confusion of responsibilities between the Departments of Health and Employment, the attitude that there was no need to add 'health' to all the other reasons for lobbying against unemployment, and the fact that 'information is scattered through a variety of disciplines'. He thereby presents his account as a balanced appraisal of the mixture of reasons why, by October 1985, it was still considered that 'we knew little' of the effects of unemployment on physical health. The risk of being identifiable as his informants so alarmed Smith's 'expert group', however, that they asked not to be acknowledged publicly for their role.

Indeed, for all the 'respectability' of having its own series in the *BMJ* being seen as a believer in the health effect of unemployment was still to occupy a controversial position. In July of 1985, within a week of each other, Norman Fowler, then Secretary of State at the DHSS, could write to Meacher: 'I would not question that unemployment may well have a negative effect on health in many cases, though by no means in all'. And Wyn Roberts, Parliamentary Under-secretary of State for Wales could reply to a Parliamentary Question by Anne Clwyd: 'I repeat that there is no direct proven causal connection between unemployment and ill health' (*Hansard* 8 July 1985. col. 703).

In November of 1986, a paper entitled 'Unemployment and health: some pitfalls for the unwary' was published in *Health Trends*, a lesser-known journal devoted mainly to health service issues, but refereed and regarded as 'respectable'. It was by an economist, Adam Wagstaff, who had recently completed a PhD under the supervision of one of the leading health economists:

Prof Alan Williams at the Centre for Health Economics at York. He threw down a challenge at the beginning of his paper: 'Contrary to what is often asserted ... the evidence regarding the impact of unemployment on health is far from clear-cut' (Wagstaff 1986c). He emphasises the 'complex methodological problems' involved and the fact that because of these complexities 'it is frequently difficult for the non-specialist to evaluate the strengths and weaknesses of research reports about unemployment and health.' He criticises Moser *et al*, for not controlling for past health in their analysis and claims that 'unemployment status at April 1971 will tend to act as a proxy ... for health status at April 1971'. In other words 'unemployed' is a sign of being in poorer health. This completely ignores the argument that if the unemployed were an 'unhealthy' group, the effect of such selection on mortality should 'wear off' over time. Wagstaff's paper was noted by the UHSG, but had no media or political impact, at least not in the 'public domain'.

Metamorphosis

The rest of the academic debate on unemployment and health in between mid-1985 and March 1987 was low key, and demonstrated a process of metamorphosis. The above examples of research findings and reports show the way in which the debate had to some extent become frozen into an opposition between approaches which emphasised explanations based on 'individual selective' factors (preexisting ill health, smoking, mental instability) and those with emphasised 'structural' factors (poverty, stigma). At this time, members of the LS team were working on a commission from the DHSS to examine patterns of social mobility amongst members of their 1 per cent sample of the 1971 census. The monograph was completed by August of 1986, and though it was never published (parts of it appeared in shorter papers and in an OPCS monograph [Goldblatt 1990]) it must have influenced their thinking on unemployment.

The ongoing work of linking up data on their sample in 1971 to the 1981 census had confirmed to the LS team that: 'Marked changes in the shape and structure of the labour force took place between the 1971 and 1981 censuses'. These changes did not affect the outcome that: 'Socio-economic disadvantage in 1971 would appear to be predictive of unemployment and ill-health in 1981' (Fox 1986).

Most of those unemployed in 1971, apart from those in the older age groups, were once again in employment ten years later. But those unemployed in 1971 had tended to be downwardly socially mobile. They were also more likely to have experienced marriage breakdown and movement from owner occupation to local authority housing. Furthermore, the children of those unemployed in 1971 were 'disadvantaged' in terms of their risk of unemployment, the type of occupations they did obtain, and the type of housing they ended up in, regardless of the social class of their fathers. The monograph ended with an expressed fear that economic change was giving rise to an 'underclass' of multiply disadvantaged families.

During this time, Kath Moser and colleagues were also working on another paper, which would update the findings of the LS to include 1981 Census data on employment status linked to mortality between 1981 and 1983. At least one of its author group felt that the message of this paper was ambiguous. It seemed, on one reading, to be a report of *lower* mortality amongst men seeking work in the week preceding the 1981 census (the 1981 'unemployed') during the period 1981–3 than had been found in the period 1971–3 for those 'unemployed' in 1971. In other ways, however, the data seemed to indicate that the experience of unemployment had greater impact on health in the 1980s than in the 1970s.

The argument of the paper was that when comparing the effect of unemployment on mortality in the years following the 1971 Census with that in the three years after 1981, three factors had to be taken into account.

- Unemployment had risen greatly, perhaps tending to make the unemployed a less 'deviant'' or 'selected' group.
- The numbers of men 'permanently sick' and 'early retired' had also risen greatly, so that those still in the labour market even if unemployed might be more highly selected for *good* health.
- The length of the average spell of unemployment was now much longer than in the early 1970s.

In the last point, a paper in the *Employment Gazette* for September 1986 (Hughes and Hutchinson 1986) had shown that the average number of weeks spent in unemployment in 1971 had been 8.4; in 1981 it was 20.5. These three factors might give rise to two opposing trends. The first two would tend to weaken any association of unemployment with mortality. The third might tend to strengthen the association. The results of the analysis duly demonstrated all three tendencies. The LS researchers adopted the strategy of comparing death rates for the years 1981–3 (all that was available at this time) with those for 1971–3. First they compared the death rates for the whole of the two three-year periods. In the period 1971–3, the SMR for men of working age at death who were seeking work in Census week 1971 was 121 (adjusted for social class). In 1981–3 the equivalent figure was 112. Neither of these SMRS is significantly different from 100 (the average for the population).

These figures were broken down by age, and mortality ratios for each of the three years were examined separately. The result of doing this made a different interpretation possible, and this is the one adopted in the paper. For younger men (15–44 at death in 1971–3, 16–44 at death in 1981–3) the SMR is 162 in 1973 and 160 in 1983. This figure, because of the small number of deaths in the younger groups, is still not significantly greater than 100. But for the group of older (aged 45–64) men in which deaths are more common, taking deaths in 1983, the SMR is 145, significantly above 100, and much higher than the SMR of 123 for men 'seeking work' in 1971 who died aged 45–64 in 1973. The effect of selection by good health into unemployment rather than permanent sickness is also more visible in the 1981–3 period. The SMRs for the older men being below 100 for the single years 1981 and 1982, but jumping to 145 in 1983, a classical 'healthy worker effect' pattern, as the text points out. The authors conclude; 'It therefore seems that for men at older working ages, the data for 1983 provide the most appropriate estimate we have of mortality among those who were seeking work in 1981'.

Adding the 145 of older men in 1983 to the rate for younger men gave an overall SMR for this year of 147. Moser *et al.* comment: 'The standardized mortality ratio of 147 at ages 16–64 in 1983 is the best measure we have of overall mortality among men who were seeking work [on census night] in our sample'. With these words they nail their colours firmly to the mast of the 'wearing off of selection effect'. Without this argument, the figures could be interpreted as having demonstrated even less of a cause for concern in the 1980s than in the early 1970s. One co-author of the paper felt, therefore, that readers and potential

publishers of the paper might well react 'So what?' Any claim to
have demonstrated a cause for concern is based on the adoption
of the 1983 figure the 'true' effect, the one visible after the effects
of health-selection into the 'seeking work' category (as opposed to
long-term sickness or early retirement) had 'worn off'. The paper
also makes reference to the team's unpublished work on social
mobility and possible 'residualisation' in the families of those
men who had been unemployed in 1971.

The paper appeared on 10 January 1987 in the *BMJ* (Moser et
all. 1987a), and provoked one hostile response. In a letter to the
BMJ, Dr B. S. Smith writing from a Midlands district general
hospital (B. S. Smith 1987), accused the LS team of having done no
more than shown that 'men who are at higher risk of ill health are
more likely to be unemployed and more likely to die.' Smoking,
he argues, echoing Cook and the economic advisers (with whom
he had no contact) could produce both the observed high rates of
lung cancer and be indicative of

> personal or personality problems which lead to alcohol
> abuse, drug dependence, and broken marriages ... Smokers
> are more likely to have road accidents, to have psychiatric
> problems, and to have been in prison ... Because they con-
> tinue to smoke, smokers would seem in general to possess
> less motivation.

In their replies (Moser *et al.*1987b, c), Moser and colleagues did
not use the argument from selection effects wearing off, rather
surprisingly. They argue that their men 'seeking work' were
selected for good health at the beginning of the study, that the
great majority of the 1981 unemployed were in steady jobs in 1971
(according to the unpublished monograph on social mobility), so
that the 1981 unemployed can hardly be seen as some sort of
deviant group. If the mortality of the larger, more socially heterogeneous unemployed group in 1981 so closely resembles that of
the 1971 unemployed, how can both effects be due to predis-
posing factors? They conclude:

> Reduction in cigarette smoking and changes in other aspects
> of lifestyle with adverse health effects are, of course, desir-
> able. However, it would seem from available evidence that
> they are unlikely to be successful in removing health in-
> equalities unless other problems associated with unemploy-
> ment and poverty are also tackled. (K. A. Moser, P. O.
> Goldblatt, A.J. Fox, D. R. Jones 1987b)

This letter is far less technical than any of this group's previous work on unemployment and health. It replies to Smith's claims about the moral characteristics of smokers and the unemployed in more political than technical terms. There seems to be nothing in the data they have presented on 10 January or elsewhere which would act as clear evidence *against* some kind of hypothesis to the effect that over the long term, 'smokers' could be the ones worst affected by recession. The one possible technical argument, that the effect of smoking on a cohort, like that of chronic illness (or indeed 'suicidal tendencies'), might be expected to 'wear off' over time as smokers (and suicidal persons) died, and that mortality in a group 'selected for smoking' would therefore not exhibit the 'healthy worker' pattern of low mortality levels becoming higher with time, is not made here. Rather, these two letters make opposing claims of a more directly 'political' kind – should health inequalities be tackled by policies directed at the behaviour of individuals or by macro-economic policies bearing on poverty and unemployment?

The tone of this letter seems to indicate the beginning of a renewed effort by the LS team to 'enrol' allies, perhaps of a new kind. Which made it all the more frustrating for them that the media response they expected to their paper 10 January did not materialise. Only a single article appeared, in *The Times* of 9 January (Prentice 1987). There were no calls to City University requesting television or even radio interviews and no other coverage in national or local daily papers or weekly journals. More galling still, *The Times* piece was the result, not of the appearance of the paper in the *BMJ*, but of a visit to the SSRU by a feature-writer in search of 'background' material for an article on a factory closure.

The question to be asked, therefore, by the researcher into the social problem process (as opposed to that asked by the dismayed participants) is why, on this occasion, unlike in 1984, the interest-groups who had once provided the information subsidy that carried Moser and colleagues' earlier paper into at least some degree of limelight did not behave the same way in 1987? Their final contribution to the debate, taking the overt stance that unemployment was more harmful to health in the 1980s and in the 1970s, received no response from writers for the quality media. It did not result in television interviews for its authors, large international conferences or even Questions in Parliament. Three weeks after

the publication of the paper, the MRC told Fox that his request for
a new programme grant of five years to continue work on the LS
had been cut to two. Shortly afterwards, the team were told that
due to the large pay rise granted academic staff by a national
wage agreement, it was doubtful whether even two more years
work could be funded by the MRC. (In the event, they did receive
two years' funding).

This is the paradox of the unemployment and health debate: as
evidence on the topic accumulated for Britain, evidence which
appeared to be more relevant and methodologically sophisticated, its impact on public debate diminished. Moser and her
colleagues' final work on unemployment and health in the LS was
never criticised seriously in any academic journal, or anywhere
else for that matter. On the contrary it was and continues to be
widely cited. Papers continued to appear sporadically in academic journals, some seeming to accept unquestioningly that unemployment damaged health, others continuing to treat it as an
open question. Perhaps for some readers what was said by participants, written in minutes of meetings, printed by newspapers
and academic journals will be enough to explain the paradox.
However, the second section of this account will turn back to the
institutional structures and social practices within which the debate took place in an attempt to offer an explanation which may
help us to understand, not just those debates which end in this
kind of twilight zone, but policy-related scientific debates more
generally.

Note

1. The papers were eventually published in book form, Smith
   (1987b).

Part Two

Authorities and Partisans

8
INTRODUCTION

At the beginning of this book no claim was made that the first section would be a purely factual account of events. It was pointed out that the account offered of the debate was shaped from the beginning by ideas as to how it could eventually be analysed and understood as a case study in the relationship between research and policy debate.

Accordingly the narrative itself has been organised roughly into 'stages' following the methods of social-problems theorists in the tradition of deviance theory. Within this framework, concepts drawn from the 'strong programme' and 'translation' perspectives in the sociology of scientific knowledge have been used to organise information on events and actions. Part Two will look more closely and analytically at some of the events and participants' accounts. There are aspects of the account which indicate rather abrupt withdrawal by some of the participants. But in Part Two we will return to look at participants' reasons for entering the debate in the first place: Why did participants enter and leave the debate in the way they did? Admittedly, funding problems faced some of the researchers between 1985 and 1987. But none of the early work which produced the three most influential pieces of research was directly funded at all. In order to understand how policy and research debates interacted, we need to know more about why knowledge claims came to be made.

Even at this stage, it will be evident that the question 'Did the research affect the policy debate and if so how?' is no longer an appropriate one. The two processes are thoroughly entwined, and the aim in Part Two of the book is to understand more clearly how this works, and to reflect on the degree to which observations from this single debate might be generalisable to others. This account of the unemployment and health debate has indicated that it is not the mere existence of research findings, or even the opinion of the academic community as to their 'quality' which ensures the entry of knowledge claims into the public sphere and policy debate. This should not be too surprising to users of the 'Strong Programme' in SSK and the 'translation' approach, as these approaches imply that entrepreneurialism is required even within scientific communities themselves before knowledge claims become facts. In order to become either 'scientific fact' or 'policy-relevant', knowledge claims need to be 'points of passage'. That is, they must attract the assent of a number of groups, a network, which will pick up and pass on the claims intact to a wider audience.

The 'translation' approach may therefore be regarded, and this is the major claim of this study, as an alternative to more conventional approaches to 'the relationship between research and policy'. The strength of the approach is that it regards all knowledge creation as essentially linked to policy debates in their widest sense. Barnes (1982) has pointed out that: 'knowledge does not have inherent implications ... scientific theories do not arrive ... with instruction books attached ... Cognitively there is no fundamental distinction to be drawn between the creation of a scientific theory and its subsequent application'. What have been called here 'social problem processes' are central to policy-making, and usually involve the making of both knowledge claims and value claims by various groups pursuing a range of interests. Each process may go on to give rise to either new facts, or new policies, or both or neither. But in many cases, it is the success of value claims in changing policy which leads to the acceptance of knowledge claims as fact, rather than the other way round. The investigator needs, therefore, to keep an open mind about the direction of influence.

In the translation approach to the social study of science, keeping such an open mind is one of the basic principles of the method (further discussed below), namely the 'principle of symmetry'. Following the principle of symmetry will produce a model of the relationship between research and policy which goes a step beyond the conventional approaches. The differences between the two can be explored starting from two recent accounts of the conventional model of the relationship between research and policy, provided by Booth (1988) and Tizard (1990).

Alternative models of the research/policy relationship

Tizard (1990) has written a comprehensive and up-to-date summary of opinions on how research influences policy, from the perspective of a distinguished research career. Drawing on the work of Carol Weiss, Tizard lists four alternative models of the relationships: linear, problem-solving, political and enlightenment. The linear model, according to Weiss, best describes the relationship between basic research in the natural sciences and technological development. Most commentators agree that this is not an appropriate model for social research. The model which sees knowledge as produced in response to policy-makers' specific needs is also dismissed: policy-makers do not in fact await the outcomes of studies before taking action (or deciding not to). The third model discussed by Tizard is the political model (which she points out may masquerade as a 'problem-solving' one), in which the policy-maker or customer commissions research which they know will support a decision to do what they had already decided upon. Under this heading falls the type of 'cosmetic' research held to be commissioned by government departments when it is expedient to be able to say 'research is being done ...' (as part of the 'loop' phases in social problem process). Lastly, Tizard choses for discussion Weiss's notion of an 'enlightenment mode': 'That is, the new conceptualisations of an issue that emerge from research trickle and percolate through to both policy-makers and the general public, challenging taken for granted assumptions and creating an 'agenda for concern' (Tizard 1990).

Finding none of these fully satisfactory, Tizard moves on to discuss why it is that some studies have impact on policy, however this impact may be conceptualised. One explanation that has been put forward is that new knowledge is more likely to be applied in policy areas where decision-making is more centralised. But Tizard, judging from extensive experience, feels this notion is thrown into serious doubt by the case of recent developments in British educational policy. Her experience also renders the idea that studies have impact because of their technical quality 'very inplausible'. She ends up proposing a model in which a series of 'gateways' are involved. This is regarded as a far more specific process than the rather 'vague concept of "Dissemination"' currently in vogue with research councils. 'For every area of social policy, there are crucial gateways through which research findings must go if they are to make an impact,' she says, of which two important examples are the quality press and the media. They also include 'ideological gateways'. She concludes: 'there has to be some degree of match between the ideology of the researcher and the guardians of the gateways'.

Booth also contrasts a linear, or as he puts it, 'purist' model and a 'problem-solving' model. The first, in his view, 'holds simply that research generates knowledge that impels action ... [and is] firmly grounded in a rational view of the policy-making process'. In the second, he gives the opinon that 'it is policy rather than theory that disciplines the research' (p. 239).

Readers may recognise in both these authors' 'problem-solving' types, the 'Rothschild' principles of the customer devising the research needs and research practitioner carrying out the necessary studies.Booth draws parallels with engineering R&D. He goes on to list the standard criticisms of these rationalistic models: that research is often used to legitimate policies which would have been implemented in any case; that policy-makers use research selectively to vindicate existing states of affairs; that research is merely decorative; that it is used to head off the need for action of any kind (p. 240). The policy-making process is, in any case, he argues not sufficiently clear cut for anyone to be able to isolate an individual who makes a final decision, and therefore it is futile to search for definitive signs of 'the research influence'.

Booth contrasts the rationalist and problem-solving models of the relationship between research and policy his own version of the *political model*, in which:

> The policy process comprises different groups, with different interests, in pursuit of different ends [and] research becomes entangled in the political debate between these constituencies (p. 244) ... For policy research to exert any influence it must inevitably be embedded in political struggle ... In this process researchers *act as partisans* for the value of their research. (p. 245 my emphasis)

Thus he adds to the picture of ideological compatibility drawn by Tizard a notion that researchers who influence policy debate are those who set out to do so.

In the early 1970s Haberer, writing from the scientist's rather than the policy analyst's point of view, lamented that:

> Politics has not become more scientific ... science has become more political ... the hierarchical structure of ... science ... with ... its large-scale institutions, ... creates varying constituencies, interest groups and organised sources of support and ... opposition, ... within ... the scientific community. (Haberer 1972)

More recently Parker (1983) has indicated the potential importance for social policy of 'the investigation of the politics of research', and Rein (1980, 1983) has called for a study of the 'interplay' between social science and social policy, rejecting notions of 'utilisation' as a one-way process. Rein proposes that:

> there are no facts [for example] about unemployment ... that are independent of the policy considerations that inform them ... the analytic concepts are themselves policy concepts ... the challenge is not linking research to policy but uncovering the latent policies which organize the empirical research. (Rein 1980)

Here in fact Rein does not perhaps go far enough along the road he has pointed out to us, in that the above suggests that 'latent policies' are not themselves shifting and open to negotiation. As Gillespie *et al.* (1979) have pointed out (as did several participants in the unemployment and health debate): 'What takes place is a dialogue with ... the information provider suggesting questions to which the policy-makers might like to find answers [because often] policy-makers themselves have not defined their need'.

Lindblom (1979) writes of the *'partisan mutual adjustment'* which takes place between experts and the parties in policy debates to arrive at both a satisfactory account of 'the facts' and a solution which will eventually be implemented. The interactive relationships discussed by Rein and Lindblom, and the 'partisan' approach recommended by both Booth and Tizard have implications for understanding research itself as tied-in with policy debates: the very 'facts' themselves may be the outcome of the overall processes of mutual accommodation between all parties, scientists included.

What these approaches all somewhat underemphasise is the micro-political activism undertaken by many scientists regardless of their policy orientations at the macro level. This additional step is most fully analysed by 'translation' theorists in the sociology of science. Latour sums up the relationship between science and its applications:

> Speaking about theories and then gaping at their 'application' has no more sense than talking of clamps without ever saying what they fasten together ... every time you hear about a successful application of science, look for the progressive extension of a network. Every time you hear about a failure of science, look for what part of which network has been punctured. (1987, p. 242)

And furthermore:

> We know that these networks are not built with homo-
> geneous material but, on the contrary, necessitate the
> weaving together of a multitude of different elements which
> renders the question of whether they are 'scientific' or
> 'technical' or 'economic' or 'political' or 'managerial' mean-
> ingless. (p. 232)

And, for 'translation' theorists, the network in question includes
all the parties to what are thought of as the 'issue communities' of
a modern polity: political parties, professions, bureaucracies of
both state and private industry. Latour gives us a graphic picture
of the process 'in action':

> before the boss [of the laboratory] enters his office, the Min-
> ister of Health is still uncertain whether or not it is worth
> investing in neuroendocrinology; the boss is uncertain
> whether or not the minister will keep the promise ... about
> funding a new laboratory; he is also uncertain as to whether
> or not ... firm promises can be made ... about [his newly
> invented substance] curing drug addicts ... It is possible that
> the ... drug addicts, the boss, the counsellors, the Minister
> and the Congressmen will all become aligned with one
> another so that, in the end, laboratory work has a bearing on
> health policy. (p. 176)

Which could be paraphrased in the following way:

> *Before the Director of the Longitudinal Study enters his office, the
> Minister for Health is uncertain whether or not it is worth invest-
> ing any more money in the LS ... The Director is uncertain
> whether any firm promises can be made that the wearing-off of
> selection can reliably distinguish between those forms of health
> inequality which are due to social conditions and those which can
> safely be attributed to unavoidable illness ... and regarded as
> beyond the scope of policy measure ... It is possible that ... the
> Director, the Minister, his Advisors, and the data from the LS and
> other studies will all become aligned with one another so that, in
> the end, the work of the LS has a bearing on social policy.*

But Latour demonstrates by a rich collection of case studies that
this possibility of alignment is a fragile one, an 'accident prone
process'. The next chapters will therefore go behind the public
statements of the controversy on unemployment and health to
look at this process. We can now look back at what happened in
the debate using all four of the principles set out by Latour and his

colleagues for studying science.

The first principle of the translation model is that the analyst should avoid 'drawing up a double entry ledger with science on one side and society on the other' (Latour 1984a). Instead, the investigator should 'follow the course of the action wherever it leads' (Coutouzis and Latour 1986). The first principle thus recommends a similar procedure to Spector and Kitsuse's method for the study of social-problem processes.[1] They add that scientists and technologists themselves do not divide society from science, but artfully negotiate the stages of claims-making process in which they are engaged (Latour 1981).

'The second principle is to 'begin with controversy' (Coutouzis and Latour 1986), that is, cases where the experts themselves disagree and are themselves (to the advantage of the observer) engaged in discussion of each others' positions, presuppositions and prejudices. If one starts from controversy and makes no presuppositions about what is fact, or even who is expert, it is found that a discussion will often 'mix experts, politicians, and the rank and file', all of whose roles must be equally attended to if the process of a debate is to be understood (Coutouzis and Latour 1986).

The third principle is that of 'maintaining symmetry' (as in Bloor 1973, 1976; Gilbert and Mulkay 1984) This is an important precaution when studying scientific controversies (whether these are obviously policy-related or not). Specifically, the principle enjoins the analyst to seek to explain both 'successful' and 'unsuccessful' claims ('true' and 'false' hypotheses) in the same terms. It consists in not assuming anything about who is right and wrong, what is 'real science' and what is 'mere politics', or even who is doing science and who is doing politics, management, business. There can be no appeal to unexplicated notions of 'rationality' or 'the outside world' to explain the success of some theories only. Nor should consideration of social or political factors be absent from the explanation of 'truth' and confined to the explanation of 'error'.

Those claims which become accepted as fact, as well as those which do not, are regarded as produced by political, econonic, social, psychological and material factors, without privileging one or the other. It is therefore not acceptable or useful to wait until we think we know what the truth really was all along, and analyse only why some people took so long to see it. It should be emphasised here that in the present study the 'outside' world, or 'nature' is not taken to be either absent or dominant in the explanation of scientific controversy. Rather, the material world or its representations in ticks on questionnaires, answers to census questions, ECG readings, computer printouts and the like is regarded by the sociologist (as by scientists themselves) as a potential ally or opponent in claims-making strategies. These inscriptions (in Latour and Woolgar's terms) are of the same importance as institutions, businesses, funding bodies, other scientists, etc. Nor is it to preclude observing that scientists (and others) judge and comment on the 'quality' of each other's work, judging some to be 'good science' and some to be 'bad science'. The principle of symmetry does demand, however, that the sociological observer be sensitive to the contextual and temporally specific nature of such judgements.

The fourth principle is that of 'explanation by association and situation'. The sociologist cannot give an account of victory or defeat except by means of the presence or absence of allies and powers at the right time and in the right place (Coutouzis and Latour 1986).

In the application of these principles to a case-study of the transfer of a technology (solar power) to a developing region, Coutouzis and Latour found that they offered great advantages, foremost amongst which was that one can 'follow controversies in hot blood, even the most bitter ones, whether they be about electric cars, gravity waves, neutrinos ... instead of arriving at the end to distribute prizes to the heroes and brickbats to the villains'.This method does not hesitate to enter the situation where there is everything to play for (Coutouzis and Latour 1986). The 'translation model' is therefore well suited to understanding cases of policy-relevant scientific and technological controversy. Rather than assuming that distinctions between what is really science and what is really politics are self-evident, we can look at the social processes which lead to definitions of 'the current state of knowledge'. Rather than struggling for the real truth about the relationship between unemployment and health we can try to understand why individuals and groups lined up on one side or the other, or sat on the fence.

First we will look at the map which lay before potential participants in the early days of the debate, in order to see what were the aims and objectives of the most active participants, and the kinds of alliances and enrolments could have appeared possible. Then we will concentrate on the scientists rather more closely to see them engaged in ongoing processes of knowledge construction, and how 'the health of the unemployed' fitted into these. Then the debate can be re-examined as a series of attempts by the different individuals and groups involved to create and hold together networks of allies, and the ways in which the fate of these attempts affected ideas about both 'knowledge' and 'policy'.

Notes

1. Latour, Callon and their collaborators extend their perspective to embrace the study of technology, by regarding the acceptance of new *artefacts* as the outcome of strategic social action in the same way as the establishment of new 'facts', see Bijker, Hughes and Pinch 1987, pp. 83–106.

9

TECHNOLOGIES OF WELFARE

The rationalisation of public health

The 'effect of unemployment on health' was placed on the agenda of policy-makers and researchers in Britain by the actions of Peter Draper and some of his colleagues at the USHP in the late 1970s. So a good place to begin an analysis of the debate is here. Why did the USHP take up the work of Brenner with such enthusiasm, playing the role of the entrepreneurs of Brenner's ideas, and, later, of the British research which claimed to show some effect of unemployment on health? What forces transformed an inside page article in *The Financial Times* in to a major academic debate? A related question which was occasionally asked, with justification, was why Brenner's work became so much more controversial in Britain than in the United States. Why did it receive the attention and political brokerage from individuals such as Draper and Scott-Samuel? The quick answer to this is that in the United States there have been Schools of Public Health independent of medical schools for many years. Public health in that country is an established technology of welfare. It has a far larger membership and a more secure prestige both as a practising profession and as an academic discipline than is the case in the UK. Furthermore, the Diploma in Public Health (DPH) is a recognised professional qualification open to those with and without medical training, to which there is no equivalent in Britain. One reason for the shape taken by the debate in the UK must be sought in the position of 'public halth' here in the mid-1970s, a period of change and uncertainty.[1]

In the 1970s and 1980s a series of profound changes were taking place in what was the beginning of the period (and again now) called public health medicine. Some of these were intended rationalise public expenditure on health, and others to produce a form of knowledge appropriate to this rationalisation.

The history of the British NHS has been accompanied from its inception by debates on expenditure. In the early 1950s, R.

Titmuss and B. Abel-Smith re-analysed figures from the Guille-baud Committee Report to show that the 'crisis' of rising costs was largely an artefact of inflation (Ham 1985, p. 19). A short period of growth in the NHS which followed Guillebaud overlapped with the adoption by British government of American style operational research techniques. These techniques, although not solely intro-duced for these reasons, continued to be used in the attempt to cope with the economic constraints which began to be more strongly felt in the mid-1970s (Butler and Vaile 1984, p. 78–9; Ham 1985, p. 93–4). In 1968, the Labour government, in the wake of devaluation, 'took a serious look at controlling the size of the public sector and converted the small steps that had followed since the 1961 Plowden Report into the powerful PESC (Public Expenditure Survey Committee) system' (Heclo and Wildavsky 1974, p. 274). During this period of administrative reform (Fry 1981), it was discovered that; 'Ministers lacked sophisticated in-formation and analysis such as that used in US programme budg-eting. The result was that resources were being allocated without much reasoned deliberation' (Heclo and Wildavsky 1974, p. 268).

The impact which this had on the Department of Health was stated by a DHSS official, H. C. Salter, at a seminar on health economics held at the University of York's new (DHSS funded) Health Economics Unit in 1970:

> One might expect during Public Expenditure Review that there should be some scientific judgement of priorities and of the merits of cutting one programme instead of another … But at present there are no means of arriving at scientific assessments … We are very conscious that in this new approach, we [Health and Welfare] may well lose in the struggle for a proper share of the national cake if we are not able to present our case more scientifically. (Salter 1972, p. 18–19)

The participation of Abel-Smith, an economist, in the early efforts of the Guillebaud Committee to identify the causes of 'cost infla-tion' in the NHS and impose 'priorities' and criteria of cost effec-tiveness and value for money acts as a reminder of the long pedigree of these exercises.

During the early 1970s there was an increasing emphasis on the need for planning, evaluation, efficiency and cost effectiveness, both in health and in other areas of public administration, in an attempt to control what had come to be seen as runaway growth in government expenditure. The emphasis on planning, in turn, gave rise to perceived needs for different kinds of information about the health and welfare of the population and the provision of services, and for new kinds of experts to collect and analyse this information. In particular, there was increasing dissatisfaction with the individual doctor's clinical judgement as the determinant of spending on health care. This opened an opportunity for other professional or disciplinary groups to make claims to a different, non-clinical form of expertise in the health field.

'Public health' and 'social medicine'

One candidate for the role of providing an appropriate knowledge base was a sub-discipline with a variety of names which can be referred to here as 'social medicine'. In the late nineteenth and early twentieth century a prominent role in public policy debate and formulation had been played by statistically-inclined doctors working in public health. As Lewis puts it:

> The term public health invariably conjures up images of the heroic nineteenth century battles to provide sewerage and clean water, led by figures such as Edwin Chadwick, William Farr and Sir John Simon. Unlike twentieth century civil servants, these men were zealots, seemingly unafraid of taking a strong stand and pursuing their own policies. (Lewis 1986a, p. 1)

This tradition of medical involvement in community health and prevention issues was a strong one in both Europe and the US. However, Lewis points out that two developments in the late nineteenth and early twentieth centuries combined to reduce the importance of the public health doctors (the Medical Officers of Health): control of the greatest threats to health in the growing towns and cities by sanitary engineering and hygienic regulation and the acceptance of 'germ theory' which allowed epidemics to be understood in terms of specific micro-organisms rather than environmental conditions more generally

One form in which the environmental public health tradition continued in the 1950s and 1960s was as a faction within the new academic discipline known as 'social medicine' (whose history is told in Watkins 1984). In 1943 J. A. Ryle, the Regius professor of Physic at Cambridge University took up a newly instituted Chair of Social Medicine at Oxford University, and before the end of the war, other chairs were set up in Birmingham and Edinburgh. In other medical schools, departments of public health either changed their titles or made other moves to symbolise their adoption of the 'social medicine' perspective. In 1947 a new *British Journal of Social Medicine* was launched, and the MRC set up a Social Medicine Unit in London under the directorship of J. N.Morris, an *eminence grise* throughout this story.

There had never been a great deal of love lost between 'social medicine' and mainstream 'public health' (Webster 1986) and little consensus as to what constituted the legitimate content of the discipline. Webster (1986) reports that: 'The pioneers [of social medicine] experienced difficulty in defining their objectives ... Furthermore, the pioneers, especially Ryle ... were regarded as radical misfits. After the premature death of Ryle his chair lapsed'. After this point, academic departments began to concentrate increasingly on medical statistics and epidemiology rather than 'the allegedly "sentimental" aspects of social medicine ... often stigmatised as the "unmarried mother" category of social problems!' (Weinerman 1951, quoted in Webster 1986). At a much later date, however, some of its practitioners were encouraging social medicine to develop:

> a theory of medicine as a practice of political reform, preserving health through the realisation of full democracy, free education, national autonomy, communal self-government ... [and] ... the prevention of morbidity through the provision of economic and social welfare ... [in which] ... doctors should play a determining role. (Watkins 1986)

By the mid-1960s, as Jefferys (1986) points out, social medicine had split into two camps. One group saw their future relationship to clinical medicine as similar to that of the (high-status) clinical pathologists. They would provide expert judgement on the effectiveness of medical procedures by the use of statistical techniques to analyse the outcome of scientific trials (of new drugs for example). In this enterprise they would work with non-medical experts such as statisticians, who would however remain in a subordinate role (rather like nurses and medical laboratory scientists). This new sub-discipline was termed by some 'clinical epidemiology'. The other camp saw the future for social medicine as the underlying discipline informing the work of the Medical Officers of Health (the Public Health doctors). This group felt there was a danger if their discipline went the way of the clinical epidemiologists. The danger was that the emphasis on prevention of disease

by analysing disease patterns and recommending changes in the
wider society would be lost, and with it most of the influence of
the sub-profession over the policy-making process. The more 'political' vision of social medicine had an obvious appeal to this
group. They were searching for ways of shifting the balance of
emphasis away from a concern with the analysis of clinical effectiveness towards field studies of the distribution of disease in the
community and its causes. And for a short period it was possible
for this group to imagine an alliance with health planners who
wanted to improve the targeting of health care provision.

The transition of a section of social medicine into 'clinical epidemiology' deserves an account of its own. It bears witness to the
persistent difficulties facing any group of 'non-clinical' practitioners in gaining a secure status within medicine. By the late 1970s, a
second group of 'clinical epidemiologists' seemed to be in the
making, who used complex statistical methods in conjunction with
clinical tests of physiological function to investigate the causation
and natural history of chronic disease. The attempt by this group
to increase the respectability of the study of disease in the community was not an easy one. But it was greatly helped by, and
built upon, the definitive work of Sir Richard Doll in discovering
the link between smoking and lung cancer (see his own account of
this in Doll 1967). This group adopted a somewhat piecemeal
strategy of building on Doll's work in a search for behavioural
factors in the causation of other kinds of common degenerative
illness – primarily 'coronary heart disease' which appeared to
have reached epidemic proportions in the UK and some other
European countries in the early 1970s. Where the 'dangerous
radicals' of social medicine had highlighted environmental and
occupational conditions, these clinical epidemiologists emphasised smoking, drinking, diet and excercise as the major factors in
chronic illness. A notion of 'stress', which had so interested Peter
Draper in Brenner's work, played an uneasy intermediate role.
On the one hand, some scientists claimed that 'stress' could be
measured by analysing the levels of certain hormones in the
blood just as clinical epidemiologists measured blood pressure,
heart impulses and blood fats. On the other, 'stress' seemed to
form a link between these more 'clinical' activities and the political concerns of social medicine by locating the cause of physiological changes in social conditions.

Questions of cost and efficiency in health service delivery had not been ignored by social medicine. Although, as Lewis points out: 'The professional organisations of public health doctors gave no indication of ... wishing to change the nature of medical practice' (1986a, p. 9). In the 1960s, some practitioners of academic social medicine had turned their attention in this direction. The most well-known results are to be found in the work of A. L. Cochrane and J. N. Morris. Both these men combined skills in statistical analysis with concern for health service organisation. Cochrane carried out pioneering work in subjecting the effectiveness of intensive coronary care units to randomised clinical trials. Morris wrote the first major British paper on the health effects of unemployment (in the 1930s) with R. M. Titmuss, Britain's first Professor of Social Administration (Morris and Titmuss 1944). In his book *Uses of Epidemiology* (Morris 1964), first published in the mid-sixties, Morris laid emphasis on the importance of measures to promote health rather than merely to deal with illness once it had occurred (an approach which came to be known as 'the upstream model'). 'Prevention' was held to be of increasing importance, in a period where the pattern of disease was seen to be changing to one where most illness was caused by chronic conditions which had long (and expensive) natural histories and were, basically, incurable.

In 1972, Cochrane's 1971 Rock Carling Lecture on 'Effectiveness and efficiency: random reflections on health services' was published as a book (Cochrane 1972). It is perhaps still the most influential book written by a doctor on the subject of health service organisation. Morris used the idea of 'community diagnosis' to refer to the need to use epidemiological techniques to monitor the state of health of a population in order to build up a picture of 'need' which would allow the adequacy of health care provision to be assessed. Cochrane's notion of 'effective' treatment was one which 'altered the natural history of disease' (for the better). *Both* concepts required the monitoring of health status outside hospitals (Acheson 1968). This was to have been part of the task of the new profession 'community' medicine (see, for example, Gill 1976, Holland 1982, Morris 1971). Public health practitioners may have become less in demand for the control of infectious disease and other traditional activities of the Medical Officers of Health (Florey and Weddell 1980, Parston 1980). However, they could seek a new role by developing links with the planning and administration of health services as part of the drive toward rationalisation of the state sector which took place in the late 1960s and early 1970s. As Lewis puts it: 'The renewed interest in "prevention and health promotion" focussed on securing healthy lifestyles for individuals ... and was prompted more by a desire to prevent people becoming hospital patients – in other words, to cut hospital costs' (p. 2).

However, the cost-cutting aspect of social medicine was not the only one. There is an important characteristic of the relationship between the 'spending departments' in British government and professional groups which gives rise to some confusion. This is that officials must face in two directions: towards the Treasury on one hand and towards their own interests on the other. As a result, officials often seem to be looking for research which may support two different kinds of aim. Although the demands to keep spending within bounds are a strong influence, no department, or for that matter, division within a department, nor branch within a division wishes to find itself without a role. A government statistician described the setting up of one study in this way:

> It wasn't quite clear why this study got resources at that particular time ... One reason may have been that it was when ['X'] Division had a crisis with the Rayner Report and funding. The Under-Secretary ... was a known friend of the Division and so he threw us some work in a time of crisis. The second [reason may have been] that they genuinely wanted to know the answer [laughter].

Internal as well as external pressures therefore give rise to a demand for research that bears witness to the existence of the sorts of social problems which a Ministry exists to deal with. Before they can be, in Manning's terms 'technically fragmented', social problems must be seen to exist. Like professionals outside government, those inside must define the wants they serve.

By 1970, it appears that at least some people within the DHSS foresaw the need to be able to make their claims against other Departments in the annual battle with the Treasury appear to be 'scientifically respectable'. The disciplines to which officials looked for expertise appropriate to their claims were both social medicine and economics. Health economics had been flourishing for some time in the United States and one of the largest health-economic studies ever undertaken in the UK was Feldstein's in the 1960s (Feldstein 1967). However, to some extent, the DHSS can be said to have further promoted the discipline, by funding the York Unit specifically to train up new members (the MSc course in health economics had its first intake of students in 1977). The exigencies of the struggle between a spending Ministry and the Treasury began to create a space into which another entrepreneurial sub-discipline could move (for an explicit debate amongst economists on this point, see Engelman 1980, Akehurst 1981). In 1970, the DHSS introduced an output budget for health and personal social services, which would routinely relate expenditure more closely to objectives (Banks 1979, p. 154). 1970 may be also regarded as marking the establishment of 'health economics' as a distinct sub-discipline in Britain centered around the York unit (Porter 1979, and for sociological observations on the work of this research group, see Mulkay *et al.*, 1987a and b).

The bureaucratisation of community medicine

Against this background of increasing anxiety over health expenditure the 1970s saw two major upheavals of health and social service organisation. As part of the 1970 reorganisation of social work (the Seebohm reforms), the Medical Officers of Health lost control of local authority social workers, who sought greater professional recognition and autonomy. The causes and effects of this are now beginning to be disputed by social historians. Margot Jefferys (1986) decribes these changes as:

> the outcome of the cleverly contrived political activities of a comparatively small number of determined individuals ... here was nothing inevitable about the the changes ... They set out to influence those with political power, they met and overcame opposition to their strategies from the two occupational groups and from civil servants.

In 1970 the Local Authority (Social Services) Act created social service departments in the major local authorities to carry out the functions of the personal social services. These large new departments were mostly headed by social workers. The status of the Medical Officers of Health (MOsH) was radically undermined by this change, and by the 1974 Health Service reorganisation. In the words of the 1972 Report on NHS management known as the 'Grey Book' (DHSS 1972), community physicians were seen as 'clinical managers'. They were granted consultant ('specialist') status so that the voice of management should have a degree of legitimacy equal to that of the high-spending hospital clinicians on the consensus teams at the various decision-making levels of the health service (for an account of the problems created by this reform, see Russell 1984, Lewis 1986b).

Community physicians therefore were absorbed back into the NHS and an ongoing debate began as to their role and domain of expertise. Were they there as administrators, in charge of medical staffing, planning and evaluation of services, or did they still have a role to play in relation to the community at large and the social determinants of health and illness? The result of reorganisation was, in the eyes of many both inside and outside of community medicine, the worst of all worlds. The role the Medical Officer of Health (MOH) in protecting and improving the environment (both physical and social) took on something of the nature of a 'myth of the golden age'. In the words of Sir John Brotherston, one time Chief Medical Officer for Scotland: 'The pioneer Medical Officers of Health had many obstacles to contend with such as primitive organisations and attitudes, but they could range freely in their concerns over the whole front of human well-being' (in Draper and Smart 1984).

Dissidents regretted the loss of the charismatic public health role, embodied in the legendary figures of Chadwick, Farr and Simon. The changes were described colourfully as 'Gotter-dammerung' by one commentator (Acton 1984), and as 'death throes' by another (Smith 1919). Some felt that community medicine had moved too far towards a purely managerial function within the hospital sector. Health authorities, unlike local authorities, are 'quangos', appointed ultimately by central government. Many within community medicine (and all who became involved in the unemployment and health debate) regretted the loss of accountability to an elected body and of the 'professional advisory role' which this entailed.

In an enlightening paper, Steven Farrow, the organiser of the Cardiff conference, ('To put social medicine back on the agenda of my department' as he remarked) gives expression to some of these anxieties and the way they related to the debate: 'Almost nothing' the paper complains, 'is known about the community's health at a local level', and bemoans the lack of a clear role for community medicine. In a statement of the Manifesto position, (though Farrow never attended UHSG meetings and did not have regular contact with the community physician members of the group), he concluded: 'The evidence linking unemployment to health is circumstantial but strong. In these circumstances, medicine ... has a duty to speak out against those policies that lead to increased unemployment' (Farrow 1983).

The uncertainty over their role was not, however, the only reason why sections within community medicine took up the question of whether characteristics of the physical and social environment, such as unemployment and other forms of social deprivation, affect health. The question was posed within a context where, as we have seen, a debate was being conducted how to reduce the consumption of hospital medicine. As part of this debate, great interest was being shown in questions about the 'determinants of health'. At this time, in Jefferys' words, there was a 'belated recognition that the NHS and social welfare services were not dealing primarily with a satiable backlog of need but with a situation in which demand was not merely always likely to exceed supply, but also one in which supply itself stimulated demand'. And under these circumstances, she continued: 'attention on both sides of the political fence and by adminstrators began to be concentrated on ways of modifying the relentless tendency for supply to increase and on improving service performance' (Jefferys 1986).

This new debate on the causes of, and solutions to, seemingly limitless demand for care seemed to give a new importance to the concerns of social medicine. The languishing discipline could hope to play an important role as the knowledge base for a challenge by community physicians to the hegemony of the high-technology, high-spending, curative branches of medicine, and thus bring its advocates into an alliance with interests within government.

This role had two faces: community physicians could concentrate on 'limiting supply' – by closing down under-utilised small hospitals for example. Or they could concentrate on lowering demand. Research in social medicine had for some time been demonstrating that the major determinants of health lay, not in clinical medicine, but outside, in the standard of living and lifestyle of the population as a whole. The foremost advocate of this position was McKeown, who occupied the Chair of Social Medicine at Birmingham University (discussed above) and his collaborators (see McKeown and Lowe 1966; McKeown 1976, 1979). An expert advisory role vis-à-vis the local authorities, who are responsible for housing, social services, environment, and education (including Health Education) was therefore regarded by an active faction within community medicine as preferable, both in terms of political structure and of the possibility of taking necessary actions to promote health. It was therefore ironic, in the eyes of many commentators on health policy, that at this of all times, the 'community' physician should be more than ever tied to management of clinical medicine.

A loosely connected faction among community physicians was forming around these discontents in the early days of the unemployment and health debate. Taking some liberty, I have referred to this tendency – a set of ideas rather than a stable group of individuals, as 'Manifesto' community medicine. The 'Manifesto' document 'Re-thinking community medicine' (USHP 1979), was produced by the USHP. Members of the USHP were the promoters, in Britain, of the ideas of M. H. Brenner. The 'Manifesto' community medicine group aimed to influence both the profession's major client, the Department of Health, and the content of their professional functions. They envisaged the use of epidemiological methods by both medical and non-medical researchers to establish both 'need' and 'outcome of care'. The resulting indicators would then be used both to plan service provision and to evaluate the performance of clinicians. Amongst their natural allies were therefore those engaged in any form of health research or information-gathering who, for whatever reason, located some of the determinants of community health levels at the 'political/ environmental' level. This group included a group of statisticians inside government departments who had promoted 'social indicators' in the 1960s and 1970s, whose role and very existence was to be threatened by administrative reviews carried out under the post-1979 Conservative government. These groups shared a vision of the use of sophisticated statistical techniques becoming available at that time to demonstrate the need for and promote 'the prevention of morbidity through the provision of economic and social welfare', to repeat Webster's words. A high priority was therefore given by 'Manifesto' community medicine and its sympathisers to questions of health inequality, as reflected in the membership of the working group which produced the Black Report: one was J. N. Morris, another Peter Townsend, a student and colleague of Titmuss.

Brenner's ideas also fitted in with notions being promoted by USHP and by the 'manifesto' group within community medicine because he was promoting the concept of a 'managed' economy, an essentially Keynesian idea, but with the addition that indicators of health should be used as well as purely economic indicators, as measures of an economy's ability to promote 'welfare' as well as 'wealth'. Brenner (whose early training had been in economics) and the USHP team shared a view that economic policies should be designed to take into account their contribution to human 'health capital' and their health costs. This potentially offered an important role to community physicians, one which some regarded as nearer to that of their forbears, the Medical Officers of Health. *Radical Community Medicine* gave expression to some of the views and ideas produced within this fragile alliance, and the effect of unemployment on health was a highly suitable topic for their attentions.

The USHP embodied many of these ideas in its work. The entrepreneurial activity of the unit was directed towards the DHSS, and, simultaneously, at the community medicine establishment' (in the words of one of its senior staff). USHP attempted to promote a far more influential role for community medicine and its practitioners within the re-organised NHS. In order to advance these claims within the medical profession, USHP and its sympathisers attempted to mobilise the anxieties of the Department of Health over excessive spending on 'high technology curative medicine', and to direct attention to the social and environmental aspects of the prevention of ill health and its associated costs (the 'upstream model'). In order to influence government opinion, they directed their ideas on the social causation of illness to the political party in power, which might have been expected to be sympathetic.

The journal *Radical Community Medicine* began to appear in 1979, the same year in which *Rethinking Community Medicine* was published. The editor of *Radical Community Medicine* became co-ordinator of the UHSG, the major pressure group in the debate. When the USHP was closed down, the UHSG effectively took up its role as the promoter of Brenner's ideas, and of the subsequent research in the UK claiming that there was a connection between unemployment and health. Scott-Samuel and Draper were old allies: in 1984 a rumour circulated that Draper had said he regarded the younger Scott-Samuel as 'his successor' (whether it was true or not, it was a plausible idea to participants in the debate).

The market for expertise

This account of developments in public health clarifies what was at first a surprising characteristic of the issue community around 'the health effects of unemployment'. This was how commonly participation in pressure groups itself seemed to constitute a form of 'professional entrepreneurialism'. The necessity to consider this phenomenon emerged from an apparently trivial problem which arose during the fieldwork for this study. When writing up and organising field notes, interview material was anonymised by assigning codes, and the intention was to give a letter to each interviewee which indicated the 'group' to which he or she belonged. It proved very difficult to decide for several participants whether to regard them as 'professional' or 'activist'. As quite often happens, a technical problem proved to be of wider significance. Two things may seem obvious by now in relation to this 'coding problem'. Firstly, that it is to be expected from the analytical perspectives adopted that these two categories would not be distinct. Secondly (this will be discussed in more detail later) that perhaps some analytical lesson should be learned from the relative *ease* with which, in this particular case study, the *researchers* could be distinguished from the activists. The innocent 'coding scheme' used in early stages was in fact thoroughly imbued with a set of assumptions about how science is done and how it feeds into policy debate (a 'double entry leger'). Because the assumptions were wrong, the coding 'did not work'.[2]

The tendency for 'expertise' and 'pressure' to become interwoven, and for the distinction between 'authorities and partisans' to become blurred may have been stronger during the late 1970s and 1980s for reasons to do with the increasing role of government in research funding. According to Hall *et al.* (1978), it is partly as a result of this (further discussed in the next chapter) that many of the institutions from which social scientists participated in health and welfare policy debates were what they (p. 60) have called 'intermediate bodies', and what Cherns (1979, p. 45–6) calls 'mediating institutions'. These are the research institutes and policy units such as the Child Poverty Action Group, Shelter and the Institute for Social Studies in Medical Care, which Hall and co-authors regard as situated between the more obvious interest groups such as trade unions and employers' organisations on the one side, and government on the other. In these intermediate bodies, of which the USHP was a perfect example, social scientists (including health-economists of more Keynesian than monetarist persuasion) collaborated with 'social medicine' academics on questions relating to health policy and the health consequences of wider social and economic trends. The short history of the USHP stands as an example of the tendency noted by Hall *et al.*: 'There is no firm boundary between research, pressure group activities and party politics. Altogether this 'intermediate' area ... probably accounts for many of the initiatives and much of the pressure for change in social policy'.

It may be that in the mid- and late-1970s, the charismatic role which some groups within social medicine and public health felt obliged to adopt in opposition to the threats posed by the 1974 reorganisation fitted well with this innovative tradition of extra-institutional social science.

The excessive separation in sociological research between 'pressure groups' and 'expert groups' is a problem in some versions of the social-problem perspective, despite the insights of Everett Hughes who reminded us in 1971 that:

> It is in the course of interaction with one another and with the professionals that the problems of people are given definition. Pains and complaints are the lot of the human (and other) species. But diseases are inventions. They are definitions of conditions and situations. Professionals do not merely serve. They define the very wants they serve. (Hughes 1971, p. 422)

A useful corrective to this tendency is offered by the work of the social historians Macdonagh (1958, 1961), MacLeod (1967) and Novak (1972) on the process of government growth and the role which science played in it in the early nineteenth century. Macdonagh (1958) proposes another variant of the 'stages model'. In his 'fourth stage' he deals with the effect of successful social-problem claims-making upon the organisation of occupational groups, and their relationship to the state. At this stage, a corps of 'officers' or 'inspectors' of one kind or another are appointed to see that the legislation is implemented. In stage five, the officers or inspectors develop their own entrepreneurial aims and interests as an emergent professional group, which helps the process along to stage six in which yet more legislation is passed and a central authority is established. Novak's contribution is to point out that the 'expertise' of the corps of inspectors or officers is not something which should be accepted or taken for granted. Rather, occupational groups enter the process in an entrepreneurial fashion, as makers of knowledge-claims, deliberately targeted towards attaining a role in what was at the time under study (middle and late nineteenth century) a growing state sector of the economy. Novak provides a succinct formulation of 'public health as a social problem' to which a medical profession in a state of change and uncertainty could offer itself as 'the solution':

> like any professional body or trade union, the medical pro-
> fession had to provide sufficient employment for its mem-
> bers ... entrance into the civil service [through the post of
> Medical Officer of Health] through the public health bu-
> reau-cracy meant much more to doctors than an opportu-
> nity to improve England's health ... For the doctors, the
> Medical Officership was a state-subsidized research grant
> which symbolized the state's need for medical expertise.

Here Novak provides a theoretical interpretation of the relation-ship between sections of a profession and departments of state which can be applied directly to present day policy processes in health and welfare. As Novak sees it, 'professional zeal' is 'a dynamic element in the course of bureaucratic growth' and in the 'growth of knowledge'. He does, however, cling to a concept of 'real' knowledge as something which is in some way 'other than' the sort of knowledge claims put forward by entrepreneurial professional groups. There is an implication in his work that professional entrepreneurialism is a slightly shady activity made necessary because no one really knew much about the real causes of disease. In this way Novak violates the principle of symmetry. This opens him (as it does sociological analysts using a social-problem perspective) to the charge of 'ontological gerrymander-ing' (Woolgar and Pawluch, 1985a, b), that is, writing accounts of phenomena as 'socially constructed' only when the author basically does not believe in them, rather than allowing for the socially-organised character of perception and understanding in both those cases which we do and do not currently regard as 'real'. But the contribution of this work by social historians on the relationship between professions and the state forms an essential link in the understanding of present-day social-problem pro-cesses and the way in which they result in both 'policy' and 'knowledge'.

A major contribution of these social historians to developing a social-problem perspective is that they remind us to investigate the ways in which social and economic change can affect the circumstances of occupational groups. Such change may give rise to a dynamic in which groups must seek redefined roles for some or all of their members. As a writer in the tradition of the 'strong programme' of SSK was later to express it: 'professional vested interests may form the middle link which connects, on the one hand, controversies about the nature of phenomena and, on the other, conflict over the availability of resources or the securing of credibility for scientist's work' (Shapin 1982). This dynamic can, in turn, have far-reaching influence upon what come to be seen as significant scientific or social problems at a specific period.

Such forces were not opaque to participants in the unemployment and health debate of the 1980s. Some did indeed regard the activities of the community physicians as somewhat self-seeking. There were two aspects to these criticisms. Some regarded them as attempting to dominate and medicalise the issue of unemployment. Others made a more subtle point. Just as civil servants are held to benefit from a quasi-symbiotic relationship with pressure groups which may spawn 'bright deas' useful to official careers, members of subordinate sub-professions may seek similar benefits. There was a steady undertone of resentment towards the medically qualified activists, which included ironic or bitter remarks that most of the serious work in the debate had been done by non-medical participants. The community physicians were regarded as a kind of 'free-loader'. Watkins said explicitly that the UHSG was intended as a 'support group' for members doing research. Although other non-medical members at various times were also doing research, it could be argued that they gave more than they received, and that expert advice of the standard offered by, for example, Westcott on economics, might not otherwise have been so readily available.[3] And while individual research projects might benefit lay members of the groups to some extent, community physician members needed to carry out studies in order to gain the Membership of the Faculty of Community Medicine, leading automatically to lucrative consultant posts.

A similar theme ran in the history of the USHP: there was a feeling that many of the ideas behind *Rethinking Community Medicine* had been originated by social scientists who would gain little thereby. What was at stake was not only professional advancement; in 1986 one participant warned another (both sociologists) against one of the community physicians on the ground that he 'went to high powered Labour Party meetings and spouted ideas he had picked up from her'. By 1987 *Radical Community Medicine*'s editorial group had been taken over by social scientists, who changed its title to exclude the term 'medicine'. These accusations can be set in the context of the routine creation of 'bright idea' factories by relationships between state functionaries and academics or activists in other spheres. However, the conflict is important, because it probably contributed to the weakness of the alliance that claimed 'unemployment harms health'. It may be significant, also, that when community medicine was reorganised once again, and posts of Director of Public Health became available to community (now public health) physicians, such interest as the sub-profession had ever shown in unemployment disappeared entirely.

Social medicine, social statistics, and economics

The links between a community medicine in search of a new role, an academic discipline in transition from 'social medicine' to 'epidemiology', and health planners and policy-makers caught between rising costs and shrinking resources can be regarded as providing fuel to the unemployment and health debate, as it did to others. This can therefore be seen as offering some help in understanding the involvement of members of one professional group in the debate. As is also normally the case, there was a mass of individual interests, quirks and other contingencies which influenced events. A particularly important example of the latter is to be found in the relationship between *Radical Community Medicine* and the Longitudinal Study researchers.

In historical terms, the OPCS, institutional home of the LS, developed from the same tradition as 'social medicine'. It is the product of a merger between the Government Social Survey (formerly under the Central Statistical Office) and the General Register Office for England and Wales. The latter might be thought of as the oldest 'government research organisation' in Britain,[4] and has its roots in the great efforts of nineteenth-century hygienists to improve the health of industrial areas. Early reformers such as Chadwick and Farr had used mortality statistics as indicators of the 'health of towns', and sought to embarrass local authorities into providing sanitation and clean water to areas where health was poor (Flinn 1965, Eyler 1979, Lambert 1963). So that it was not only public health doctors who looked to the nineteenth-century public health reforms as a high point of their influence, but also those whose job it is to provide the vital statistics on which reformers' claims were based.

There were several leading figures in nineteenth-century public health reforms who were either not practising clinicans (such as Farr) or not medically-qualified at all (such as Chadwick). Whereas public health doctors could deplore the overwhelmingly higher status accorded their clinical colleagues in late nineteenth-century medicine, for statisticians a historically important role for the profession as a whole was in danger of disappearing if the gathering of social indicators was to be wound down. This sense was greatly exacerbated by the Rayner reviews and the threatened cuts in OPCS staffing and funding. These fears, and the potential of an alliance between social statisticians and 'Manifesto' community medicine, can be exemplified by the role played by the Radical Statistics Group (a sort of 'Manifesto' social staticians' group) in setting up *Radical Community Medicine*. Although no members of the LS team were actively involved in the group, its involvement in the early days of opened up a channel of communication.

As a result, during 1983–4 – a period of relatively intense political activity in Whitehall around the health consequencies of unemployment – Scott-Samuel conducted a lively correspondence on health inequalities with the director of the LS programme and the Social Statistics Research Unit at City University, John Fox. The two did not know each other well, but agreed on the importance of a paper by one of the government economists involved in the unemployment and health debate, Jon Stern, which appeared in the *Journal of Social Policy* in 1983. Stern's paper showed by means of a mathematical model that it was theoretically possible for most of the inequality in health between the social classes in Britain to be attributed to the failure of those with adverse prior characteristics (Stern 1983a) to take part in the widespread upward social mobility which took place during the postwar years (Goldthorpe *et al.*,1981). In their correspondence, Fox and Scott-Samuel shared a concern that the explanation of inequalities as being due to selection and selection alone would give inequality the appearance of being 'one of the laws of nature and therefore beyond our control'. Such an interpretation of health inequalities would, it is implied, leave little scope for either the practice of community medicine or the use of 'social indicators' of which Fox was one of the leading practitioners, in policy fomulation.

The LS team had no regular contact and certainly no involvement in the activites of the UHSG. But one result of the mutual interest of Fox and Scott-Samuel in the causes of health inequalities was that the latter was aware of the work which led to the 1984 LS paper (Moser *et al.*, 1984), so that the UHSG was in a position to carry out a successful 'information subsidy' as we have seen.

Here may be found a key to the 'interest-maps' being constructed by 'Manifesto' community physicians and social statisticians which had led both men into the debate on the health of the unemployed. Genetic determinism, and this was one sense in which the 'prior characteristics' described in Stern's paper could be read, leaves little space for a reformist practice of public health. Theories of inequality drawing upon eugenic ideas ('the survival of the fittest') therefore make life difficult for a statistical practice oriented towards public health as one of its client professions. The basis for the alliance between 'Manifesto' community medicine and the LS group was not centrally based on concerns to do with the health of the unemployed. The basis was a mutual interest in promoting a social and environmental rather than a genetic or individual-behavioural interpretation of the distribution of health and illness.[5]

Added to this 'technical interest' (in the terms used by the Edinburgh school of SSK) was a related 'technical interest' in a more literal sense, of the statisticians. In order to increase efficiency and effectiveness or indeed to establish these criteria at all as part of what a health service ought to be doing, many had been arguing for some time that it was necessary to develop indicators of need for, and outcome of, health care (Acheson 1961, Acheson 1968 *op. cit.*, Butler and Vaile 1984, p. 127–8). It was argued by some that community surveys using clinical measures of disease with longitudinal follow-up, or at the very least 'data linkage' (as proposed by Acheson), enabling individuals to be followed in and out of the health system, are necessary in order for such aims to be satisfactorily accomplished. Advances in computing and statistical methods were making possible forms of data linkage, and ways of analysing the resulting information, not just on groups but on individuals. Both academics and administrators involved in the unemployment and health debate commented on these issues and to some extent the design of the LS itself embodied these ideas. Such exercises would have provided valued roles for practitioners of social medicine and social statistics as producers of knowledge, with public health doctors active in policy making as their client group.

Appropriate knowledge?

The idea of using the latest techniques in information handling and data analysis to improve the efficiency of health planning and provision by establishing criteria of need and evaluating outcomes of health care would hardly seem contentious.[6] However, as the producer of appropriate knowledge for health planning in the late 1970s and 1980s, an environmentally oriented social medicine was faced with a problem: in the political and economic climate of the time the appropriateness of both the knowledge and its applications was highly doubtful, for two reasons. One was that the cost of clinical (i.e. including 'objective' measures of health such as blood pressure, lung function, etc.) field studies to establish levels of need was so great (Butler and Vaile 1984, p. 127–8). The other was, as Heller (1978, pp. 68–79) points out,[7] that the discoveries of such exercises might themselves cause political embarrassment, giving ammunition to those who continued to call for greater public expenditure on health and welfare. In defiance of the theory of 'supply stimulating demand' for health care, surveys of health needs in the community using objective measures revealed as a sizeable 'clinical iceberg' of untreated illness (Last 1963, Morrell and Wale 1976, Hannay 1979, Scambler *et al.*, 1981). Planners needed to know about population health status, the longer-term outcomes of various forms of hospital treatments and so on, and yet this form of knowledge threatened to be, in public expenditure terms, potentially as explosive as in-vitro fertilisation, organ transplantation, dialysis and other expensive forms of treatment advocated by the clinical specialities. It was not so much a technically as an administratively infeasible exercise. As one Scottish health planner, T. Drummond Hunter, put it to me: 'It is difficult to give advice to government if the advice you are giving is not what they want to hear … there is a perpetual conspiracy here to tell people at the top what they want to hear'. And the way this 'conspiracy' worked, he pointed out, was via the reluctance of civil servants who commissioned studies from scientists to be the carriers of unwelcome messages to their superiors, for fear of 'conveying the impression that he [sic] is "unsound"'.[8] So professionals and researchers walked a very fine line here when constructing 'the health of the community' as a social problem to which they could offer the answer.

An additional problem, as seen by Prof Donald Acheson, (later Sir Donald, who was to become Chief Medical Officer at the Department of Health in the late 1980s), was that of 'departmental boundaries'. In a paper entitled 'Social and medical statistics' in 1968 (*JRSS* Series A, vol.131, pp. 10–28) he commented that the prospect of regular reports on 'survival rates, operation rates, readmission rates ... which trace [patients'] course wherever they are re-admitted ... and] rates of return to work according to condition and type of treatment' had proved infeasible. Once again the real difficulties were no longer technical, but political:

> Record linkage is concerned with bringing together data about persons across departmental boundaries ... and each department sees fit to take a departmental view, which in the nature of the problems means a defensive negative view against change even when this may be in the general interest ... At the moment, alas, the departmental barriers are up and the trenches are manned. (p. 12)

The delicate position of 'social medicine' in the late 1970s and 1980s has also been commented on by Kogan and Henkel in their comprehensive account of the workings of the Rothschild structure in DHSS-funded research. Kogan and Henkel see problems in the collaboration between government and scientists as common or even routine. They point out that, at this time, epidemiology was by no means free of its historical association with 'sentimental' social medicine ('unmarried mother problems' and/or 'dangerous radicalism'), and was: 'moving from a position in which the nature of evidence and measurement and the choice of methodology were undisputed into one where ... value issues are coming to the surface (p. 20). This fact, in these authors' view, made funding of epidemiological research on the 'customer-contractor' basis increasingly problematic for a major client, the DHSS.

We must not forget that, as Lewis has pointed out for the inter-war period, in the 1970s and 1980s community medicine as a whole (the 'establishment', represented in the Faculty) laid no particular claim to intellectual hegemony over the discussion of health policy. The profession' s mainstream was content to rest upon the assurance of the medical closed shop – by decree, no lay person was eligible to become a consultant in community medicine. There was nothing inevitable in the adoption by a group within the sub-profession of a 'social/environmental'; model of the determinants of community health. By advocating such a perspective, the 'Manifesto' group was taking a major risk. There were other groups within the sub-profession which happily adopted health economics as the appropriate basic discipline. And in many ways, the latter was the line of least resistance, as it allowed community physicians to play the far less threatening role of operational research analysts with a clinical training. Economists could provide them with estimates of the 'value of health' to individuals which were perfectly usable when deciding service priorities. For example, Culyer suggests that: 'Health care is of infinite value to none of us – we smoke and drink and eat in ways that diminish our health and life expectancy ... All our daily behaviour denies that we value health infinitely' (Culyer 1976, p. 5). And Gravelle and Backhouse state firmly that: 'The health of a population is determined by decisions taken by individuals in their capacities as voters, consumers, workers, employers, health service employees or government policy-makers' (Gravelle and Backhouse 1987).

At the time of the debate, work within government departments provided a major market for the skills of both economists and statisticians. However, the work of the economists may be regarded as including a form of 'management of an economy'.[9] That of statisticians, in contrast, was more in the nature of 'management of a population'. The different technologies involved in these two different kinds of management both influenced and constrained what could or would be adopted and offered to client groups as either a 'problem' or a 'solution'. Put somewhat crudely, there was a knowledge-claim:

'Inequality' (social or medical) is a result of the 'unfitness' or 'lesser health endowment' of a section of the population. This unfitness is either inherited or acquired in early childhood (due to poor parental skills), or the product of a mixture of both influences. Therefore, differences in health or life expectancy between groups with different experiences of adult life should not be attributed to those experiences (work, income, unemployment).

This had been proposed by various researchers over a very long period of time (for an account see Jones 1986). It was reflected, for example, in Illsley's much-respected work on perinatal mortality carried out in the 1950s. Jon Stern's work on health inequality could be seen (as it was by Fox, for example) as putting forward this type of argument. This knowledge-claim came to be seen as a potential resource by policy-makers who took a counter-Keynesian stance. A good early example of this was Sir Keith Joseph's notion of 'transmitted deprivation'.

An opportunity for 'enrolment' was therefore presented to economists working with ideas of a 'human capital production function'. Although many economists would not regard it this way, there is a possible translation of human capital theory, espoused at least transitorily by several economists prominent in both the unemployment and health and the health inequality debates (Stern 1982, 1983b; Gravelle and Backhouse 1987, see also the references given above to the work of le Grand (1987) and Illsley (1986) himself on health inequality), which allows the theory to regard social position as the result of individual characteristics and 'free choices' (for example, to invest in education, exercise or a healthy diet). Individual economists may later have abandoned this interpretation, but during the most politically heated period of the unemployrnent and health debate, much of the evidence presented here seems to indicate its importance.

For many in the Faculty of Community Medicine, however, the alliance with economists, though perhaps convenient in the short term, posed a threat to their longer term viability. If, instead of social and environmental conditions, the 'determinants of health' were to be accepted as individual factors such as consumer behaviour, and inborn psychological and physical 'health endowment', then there might be (as Mackenzie, 1981a has suggested was the case in the early twentieth century public health debates, and as Fox warned Scott-Samuel in 1984) even less intellectual space for any form of community medicine. Because economists can deal far better with individual consumer behaviour (which is, after all, part of their traditional business) and clinicians with genetic defects. As a result, the 'Manifesto' group could plausibly argue that community medicine would be wise to seek to develop an approach which stressed 'the environment', and in this sense, the 'Manifesto' group, whilst often in conflict with the mainstream of the sub-profession, must also be regarded as occupying its leading edge. And in so far as community medicine was the 'customer' for so much of the activity of vital and social statisticians, these changes in professional ideology drew the scientists' concerns along behind.

Notes

1. The sub-profession known as 'community medicine' during the period of the debate has now reverted to its older title 'public health'.
2. This is one example of the 'hardness' of qualitative data. It is sometimes assumed that qualitative data is somehow 'softer' and more easily manipulated than quantitative. In the course of this study I was constantly faced with a definite tendency of my data to kick back in no uncertain terms, which left the feeling that any researcher wishing to have easily manipulable material should stick to statistics.
3. Westcott was not, to my knowledge, one of those who ever voiced these criticisms.
4. There are separate register offices for Scotland and Northern Ireland; OPCS only extends to England and Wales.
5. Although this is one possible reading of such work, as for example in Himsworth (1984) the 'eugenic' argument is not the one intended by Stern. His point was that if we take there to be a normal distribution of ability in the population, those 'left behind' at a time of high rates of mobility are bound to be those with relatively lower amounts (i.e. further to the left of the distribution). He had intended to make this clear in a final section of the paper which dealt with policy its implications. As he was employed by a government department at the time, he was advised to remove this section.
6. In the late 1980s the Department of Health was once again busily carrying out and commissioning work on these topics, and on improved methods of information management made possible by the computerisation of the National Health Service Central Registry and of many general practices.
7. Heller was an early member of the Radical Stastistics Group.
8. However, that this is not a phenomenon solely of the civil service under Thatcher is witnessed by Opie's (1968) lament over attempts to integrate economic advice into the policy-making process under Wilson.
9. This was not, of course, applicable to market oriented economists.

10

CONSTRUCTING THE OFFICIAL RESPONSE

If we regard Brenner's advent and the response of the media, politicans and pressure groups as the 'first stage' in the process of constructing the health effects of unemployment as a social problem, the 'second stage' began with an official response to the impact of Brenner's work. Because of the effectiveness of the USHP promotion of Brenner's ideas, and the availability to opposition MPs and journalists of 'dramatic events' such as suicides of unemployed people, there was some pressure for a swift response. This consisted of ministerial statements buttressed by work done by economists at Queen Mary College and the LSE. The official response is interesting not only for what it did but also for what it did not contain. Economists are only one disciplinary group with members inside government departments, and yet in the official response to the claim that unemployment harmed health it was the economists who played a very dominant role. To see how this happened, we need to look more closely at the different position of economists, sociologists and statisticians in government departments, at the evolution of research within government departments in the 1970s, and at the way way in which 'pressure' is routinely dealt with.

Social research under the 'Rothschild system'

By the late 1970s, a great deal of the research used in policy-making was either produced or commissioned by government departments themselves. Hall *et al.* date from the mid-1960s the feeling that the information needed for planning and policy making should be produced in this way. During the 1970s, according to Hall *et al.*:

> we ... witnessed ... a major shift in the relative positions of independent and [governmental] departmental research ... Government departments are now well provided with the kinds of data and expertise needed to counteract a challenge

from an outside body, should they so wish. They are also in a better position to influence the type of research being conducted outside government. (Hall *et al.* 1978, p. 79)

As early as 1956 the Guillebaud Report on the costs of the NHS recommended the setting up of a Research and Statistics Department in the Ministry of Health and thereafter the number of statisticians and economists in the department increased rapidly (Klein 1982, p. 389). Between 1965 and 1975 the number of professional statisticians employed in government increased from around 200 to 500. The Government Economic Service was set up in 1965. The DHSS, DoE, the Home Office and the Department of Employment all established their own small social research units (Bulmer 1982, p. 131). But members of different disciplines are not deployed in the same way. The statisticians, although dispersed around the various departments, have their own Central Statistical Office (CSO), part of the Cabinet Office (Moser 1973). In a similar manner, the Economic Section of the Treasury presides over the work of economists in the various branches of government. Members of both disciplines therefore have 'professional' leadership placed high in the civil service hierarchy (at Second Permanent Secretary level, see R. Walker, 1987, p. 149), and centrally directed mechanisms for training and career development. Both statisticians and economists can enter on a 'career grade' the equivalent of 'Principal' (Grade 7) and benefit from the 'fast stream' which replaced direct entry to the administrative principal grade.

Research units within government departments hold an ambiguous position, and working in such an environment may entail a particular type of career strategy for researchers, as explained by Prince (1983):

> Most policy planners and researchers realise and accept that their work methods and advice must relate to the client's needs and their ... political context [...] the planning machinery must keep close to ministers exploring, among others, options that reflect their known views (pp. 133–4) [...] policy units in British government operate in a market where they obtain work or permission to conduct work from other officials and attempt to sell their products of advice and research. (p. 143)

Social scientists usually work in specialist research or policy units headed by a professional or scientific civil servant at the under-

secretary level. The Social Research Branch of the DHSS was one
such unit. Prince comments that, in general:

> Operating within regular government hierarchies means
> units have had to adjust to the administrative culture of
> public organisations, with its concern for risk avoidance, the
> short term and the practical. This context delimits the plan-
> ning and research functions, making them specific to a par-
> ticular set of legislative and administrative concerns. (p. 117)

Bulmer (1982) goes further. He feels that the constraint of 'political soundness' does not only enter into the career considerations
of researchers working inside government. As central departments took on more information-generating tasks, they also acquired a more important role in the funding of external research.
After the Rothschild reforms in 1971, a 'major change in the philosophy and organisation of social research' followed:

> The evolution of this structure of government support for
> social research ... places considerable power in the hands of
> departments to influence the direction taken by social research
> The requirement that research should be related to an ...
> identified policy concern of a department serves to bind
> social research increasingly to *current* interests of *specific*
> departments. It then becomes more difficult to develop
> research which deals with a problem that cuts across depart-
> mental boundaries. (pp. 143–4)

Prince (1983) points out that 'policy planners and researchers
choose work topics that have senior official support and can be
implemented...' Criteria which government researchers (and, if
Bulmer is correct, increasingly outside researchers too) must take
into account when deciding which topics to pursue include: 'political implications, administrative feasibility, ("quickies", "the
unit can do it", avoid cans of worms, anticipate issues, and
develop a distinct domain [i.e. one which a unit can claim as its
exclusive territory].' (p. 151) The relevance of this analysis of the
position of various kind of 'expert' within government departments to the present study is reflected in the comments of two
other civil servants. As one administrator explained: '[Unemploy-
ment and health is] not clearly focussed in terms of departmental
responsibilities ... in organisational terms it doesn't make sense,
so there's a bit of ad-hocery about'. And according to another:

> Unemployment and health is not at all a good example of
> how things can work together constructively. In fact, it's a

particularly bad example ... In 1980, ... there'd been a lot of discussion – it did have a group of administrators who were concerned with ... issues right across the department[1] ... policy responsibility for that work would have lain with a planning department which had some of the most competent administrators around ... so it had, beavering away at it, some of the best junior administrative minds ... Unfortunately the ... impetus and expertise got shifted in the department because the policy group got radically changed and key staff moved on. So now there is no policy location for it.[2]

In any case:

although ... unemployment and health was a very interesting intellectual problem, and we got hooked on it ... what could the DHSS *do* about it? The problem was so enormous, and not in our remit. Unemployment and health is a hybrid ... it runs across two departments, two areas of responsibility. These issues that cross the pattern of organisational structures are much more difficult to handle successfully. It doesn't have an easy place in any client group oriented structures or service structures.

Leaving aside the problems involved with any possible tendency to 'short-termism', civil servants themselves felt that having research divided up according to departmental responsibilities could be a handicap, especially (as expressed above) in dealing with such a topic as 'unemployment and health'.

The research carried out within the DHSS which influenced the debate on the health of the unemployed, the Cohort Study, was carried out by the Department's Social Security Research unit. This small unit was, until 1980, located within the Statistics and Research Division. In 1980 the unit was moved into the Office of the Chief Scientist (OCS). Researchers felt that this move had not changed the type of work they did. It was felt that

Social security has always been backward on research ... The conduct of social security policy doesn't have a research base, there is no research based profession involved ... Health is different ... the Department went to town on research. When the Secretary of State set up a Research Board in the late 1960s, it got itself organised and had useful links with policy divisions.

The social security research budget had always been rather small. On the other hand, there had been a Social Security Research

Policy Committee to co-ordinate the needs of policy customers even before the Rothschild reforms. Unlike the similar Research Liaison Groups which were set up post-Rothschild to deal with separate health policy areas (as described in Rayner 1977) the SSRPC dealt with all areas of policy. As a result: 'it had at one time more than six Under-Secretaries on it ! This made it rather grand and hard to get together ... The SSRPC didn't make decisions on projects at all. It was too grand for that'.

After the reorganisations of 1979–80 the social security research budget became part of the far larger health budget. The 'customers' for the unit's work were, as before, various policy divisions. This made no difference to the perception, throughout the time of the conduct of the Cohort Study and the debate in which it became enmeshed, that the question of the health of the unemployed was problematic because:

> it straddles two sides of the Department [even though] ... we now [1986] have a Central Policy Unit – it's called something else now, it's impossible to keep up with all these new names – ... Part of its task is to pick up things which *do* cross the Department, at least I think so.

This could be a reference to the Policy Strategy Unit of the DHSS which had been given such a remit, and had presumably taken up the issue of unemployment and health precisely because it crossed departmental boundaries and required a wider perspective. Therefore it met Prince's criterion in that 'the unit [and in this case perhaps only the unit] can do it' (for a discussion of the history of policy planning units, see also Blume 1987, pp. 80–84). PSU closely matches Prince's account of an entrepreneurial policy or research group, concerned with its own 'organisational survival'. It was described as 'close to ministers ... top-level special initiatives unit, very small, full of high-flyers ... very high-profile in its time'.[3]

But we have to remember that, as an administrative civil servant pointed out bluntly, 'governments are not in the business of adding to the stock of knowledge', despite the fact that a problem might be fascinating to individuals. From which it can be seen that unemployment and health was always finely balanced in its chances of being taken up as a legitimate topic for research. In terms of cost, feasibility, the 'can of worms' criterion and the distinct-domain criterion, the issue was a loser. Pure intellectual fascination fits neither the practical ethos described by Prince nor the post-Rothschild official commissioning process. The perception of a need for research on the health effects of unemployment was, however, constantly heightened during the period between 1979 and 1982 by both media reactions and questions in parliament. Response to this kind of pressure was seen by government researchers as the 'front-line work' to which they must attend if necessary to the detriment of longer term projects. At a time of reductions in civil service personnel, 'There just is now much less time for things that are not in the front line of the Department's work like the House of Commons and the media. This is what the Department is for and that has kept people overstretched'.

Questions and answers

In the story of the unemployment and health debate, questions from Members of Parliament were seen by participants to have played a role in the process by which the health of the unemployed came to be seen as a 'social problem'. The importance of Parliamentary Questions (PQs) in the day-to-day functioning of public servants, and the extent to which the need to answer them shapes their longer-term concerns is little discussed, although Butler and Vaile (1984, p. 100) point out that the DHSS receives 5,000 each year. Within the health-policy making community, it was common knowledge, and regarded as more or less routine, if not something to be advertised, that pressure groups, such as the Maternity Alliance for example, 'briefed' MPs to ask questions on certain topics, sometimes advised in turn by research groups seeking to improve the chances of funding for some project concerned with the same topic. This practice was referred to as 'planting a PQ'. Stories were told of the friendly or 'tame' civil servant who would help to frame a question 'correctly', that is, in such a way that it could not be evaded by saying that the information was not available or too expensive to produce. The benefit to an MP of allowing him or herself to be 'used' in this way was that s/he would be noticed, and noticed as capable of carrying out well directed probes of government policy. This is part of the career strategy of the parliamentary politician. Like journalists, however, MPs must work across a broad range of issues and have not the time (if the inclination) to get on top of complex technicalities. In other words, MPs also benefit from contact with members of pressure groups, including activist researchers, who can provide 'subsidised' information. The desire to be 'noticed' also meant that a question on the effect of unemployment on health might be asked as part of a whole string of others dealing with various aspects of health policy. For MPs, as for academics, unemployment and health was just one of many possible means to an end.

The civil servants whose job it was to answer PQs (Grade-7 officials or, in the old parlance, 'Principals') usually mustered and collated the necessary information from a variety of sources, including economic advisers, statisticians and other professional advisers. Some officials seemed rather ambivalent about PQs. They certainly have 'nuisance value', and yet they were seen as a necessary part of the democratic process. As one remembered:

> Sometimes there are very important issues revealed and raised through PQs. There are a proportion of PQs that are hard to deal with. You've got all the rest of your workload on top of this. Some of them seem to be a sort of knee-jerk response to something that appeared in the *Daily Mirror*. Some of these MPs put down 13 or 14 at a time. It is a necessary evil.

Although PQs can be useful to the careers MPs wishing to be noticed and/or to lay a special claim to one area of expertise, some questions seemed to lower civil servants' opinions of MPs, to the point where an administrator or economic adviser who was in sympathy with the aim of the question could feel 'able to write it better myself'. The problem of the collaboration between administrative and 'expert' civil servants could be highlighted by a PQ. As one put it:

> This is a classic illustration. Someone from the Actuaries Department once worked for me. He was perfect at doing these sort of totally neutral, objective appraisals. But he could not bring himself to carry out the necessary work for defensive briefing, ... [Interviewer: Is that really true, then, that you have to play to this sort of script? You make it sound like "Yes, Minister".] Your first job is to defend your Ministers from making fools of themselves..You don't actually *lie*, of course. The written PQ is the classic example of how to avoid telling the truth without lying, if you like.

On the role of the PQ in the unemployment and health debate more specifically, one DHSS official at least felt that such use of Brenner's work had:

> made the Department prick up its ears. I don't know that

there was any departmental activity [on unemployment and health] before Brenner's work appeared. These analyses of Brenner's did lead to PQs being asked. It's that sort of thing that quite often happens – either a piece of research or something a pressure group does.

However, another official told me that a different criterion was used when judging how accurately a question had to be answered when it originated from 'outside':

There are different stages – for example: 'wouldn't it be nice if—?' which could come from a PQ or an 'outsider' report. For these, it's not too high on the policy agenda, so you work with broad orders of magnitude. If it's something that starts motoring and becomes a political option, then you have to get your data sorted out and do a proper analysis.

There was seen to be a distinction here between the roles of economic advisers on the one hand and those of statisticians and actuaries on the other. The latter would only be brought in once a proposal (whether it originated inside or outside of Whitehall) had given rise to a real option for policy change. Economic advisers, on the other hand, were a good source of rapidly produced estimates which might have wide margins for error, but could be used in the sort of rapid-response mode required for answering PQs. Ultimate responsibility was seen, however, as lying firmly with the administrator and not with any of the 'experts': 'I might ask … for information, but I'd stitch it together myself. We don't let the professional support groups have responsibility for PQs – only the administrators do that kind of thing'.

Administrators will have three to five days to 'get an answer together'. In the case of oral PQs, a further challenge to the administrator's skills is presented by the threat of 'supplementaries'. In this case, 'The trick is to be able to guess what the follow-up questions are going to be. This is a test of your quality, whether you can do this'.

The Parliamentary Question, then, plays a role in the career strategies of both MPs and civil servants. In most cases, the asking and answering of PQs seems to be seen as a sort of ritual which tests the 'quality' of contestants, and which can also be a first attempt to put an issue onto the political agenda, or to return it there. On the side of research professionals in government departments, quick briefing in response to or anticipation of PQ is work which is both resented and necessary. Like their peers in academic environments, social scientists inside government departments (regardless of discipline) prefer to work on longer term projects which will produce substantial outputs of scientific merit in the form of papers and books. There are many examples of such work such as the CS from the DHSS, the Women in Employment and Workplace Industrial Relations studies, and the highly regarded Research Paper series from the Employment Department. On the other hand, 'briefing' and other such 'quick and dirty' work demonstrates the utility of research professionals to the departments which employ them.

The economists role

What participants' own accounts of official reactions to 'pressure' show in these accounts is another important element in the shaping of the debate: the role played by economic advisers. Althought the CS was carried out by the social research professionals in the DHSS's Social Security research unit, the single paper using Cohort data (Ramsden and Smee 1981) which had most impact was written by two economists. Another economic adviser whose work had an even greater impact, Jon Stern, had been closely involved with the CS although his influential papers used other sources of data.

Economists outside government departments also played an vital role, as discussed above. At a time of conflict and change in the area of health policy, an energetic and entrepreneurially inclined group of 'health economists' took the opportunity to make a claim to provide the intellectual foundations for a drive to rationalise the provision of health and social services (Mulkay *et al.* 1981a and b; Ashmore *et al.* 1989). Economists' traditional relationship to government put them in a strong position. Economists hold a unique position within the British Civil Service (Booth and Coats 1978; Cairncross 1968, 1970; Sharpe 1978; C. Smith 1987). Despite the presence of members of other numerate disciplines such as statisticians and actuaries in British political administration, the economic advisers played a key role at the point in time when health economists outside government were launching their claim to a voice in health policy-making (Bulmer 1986, p. 29, p. 200, p. 292; Bulmer 1987, p. 16). Booth (1988) describes one of the factors making for economists' protected position when the Rayner reviews led to cuts in other government professional functions as the presence of:

powerful consituencies of users [of economic information]
... It is [the] lack of political muscle that largely accounts for
the relative underdevelopment of social statistics ... They
have too few friends in the right places. The result is that
economists have established almost a stranglehold on policy
analysis inside government. (Booth 1988, p 80)

This strikingly echoes Latour's emphasis on the importance of
networks ('every time you hear about a failure of science, look for
what part of which network has been punctured').

Economists' position of influence was described to me by civil
servants who became involved in the unemployment and health
debate. One attributed the success of the economic advisers to their
ability to 'sell their wares', and 'good leadership'. This administrator explained:

It depends on the issue, whether I use economic advisers.
But it also depends on the individuals involved. If I know
that [a highly-thought of economist] is responsible for something, then I use the EAs [Economic Advisers]. But if there
is, say, a statistician that I trust, then I'd use him, if he could
do it. I need to consider questions like 'If I need a quick-and-
dirty on this one, will they stand on their professional pride
and refuse to do it?' How do these people prove themselves?
It's their *utility* that is the crucial thing ... I would say that in
this Department the economists are now head and shoul-
ders above the statisticians in the ways people like me use
them ... They deliver ... What I look for is perspective –
breadth – and not being tied within one's own discipline.

And another commented:

We use the economists' and actuaries' advice a lot ... I'm not
sure where they overlap, myself ... We also have to be aware
of their professional jealousies ... Generally – can I be frank?
– the economists are better at giving answers. The actuaries
want to take over the whole policy question. I get the impression the actuaries don't feel like civil servants at all. The
EAS see the problems WE have in the way that WE [admin-
istrators] have them ... they can even anticipate the sorts of
things we are going to ask before we do!

One economic adviser felt that: 'Being aware of (and trained to
recognise) trade-offs is a big weapon' in the battle for professional
survival in the civil service. This is because; 'It provides the basis
for being able to take an *apparent* problem and then to identify the

actual problem which may or not be the same thing'. An ex-adviser cautioned, however, that the position of EAs in the DHSS and DE in the 1980s should not be taken as universal. In these two departments;

> there are a sizeable number of economists who are used quite a lot and quite well by Ministers and administrators. There are other Departments (e.g. the Home Office, Defence, and to a lesser extent the DES) ... [which] ... have very few economists. There are some other Departments, which I won't name where there are quite a lot of economists but which are generally reckoned to be graveyards for economists. Apart from ... the Treasury, DTI and DE ... the economists' influence is always provisional and can easily be lost.

Economists themselves did not, perhaps, feel the same sense of hegemony which is attributed to them by some commentators. Like the health economists, government advisers saw a need for entrepreneurialism.

Health economists shared the view of the classical commentators such as Morris and Cochrane that problems about the allocation of resources to the health sector would not be solved by 'clinical management' alone, but only by strategies which extended over wider areas of social life. They claimed that health service planning and health policy could be better carried out by economists, because it does not require clinical training, but rather a greater sophistication in operational research techniques. They also believed that the wider questions of 'the determinants of the distribution of health and health-related behaviour in the community' (which they refer to by the economists' technical term, 'production functions'[4]) could be more fruitfully discussed in terms of the use of models of consumer utilities to determine the 'value of health' than in terms of the social and environmental causes of ill-health.[5] For example in 1987, one participant in the unemployment and health debate put it:

> as economists we hope we may be forgiven for venturing in where other disciplines have, perhaps wisely, refused to tread. Our justification, or plea in mitigation, is that the investigation of the determinants of population health is in many ways akin to the estimation of production functions ... Economists have considerable ... experience with the estimation of production functions. (Gravelle and Backhouse 1987)

And an example of the confidence with which the claims-making activity of health economics was pursued in this period is provided by Culyer (1976):

> Economic analysis of health service problems is ... no game for amateurs. The quack economist is no less a threat to society than the quack doctor ... [because] below the surface lies a vast body of highly technical, mostly mathematical work in the learned journals and scholarly monographs, ... Medical policy-making has been lumbered for long enough with a baggage train of ... amateur ideologues, amateur doctors ... and amateur economists. (p. 9)

Health economists had little interest in developing (or re-capturing) a more general political-advisory role, similar to that of the nineteenth and early-twentieth century MOsH, centred around the physical or socio-political 'environment'. As we have seen, economists were well-entrenched within the existing structure of (at least some) government departments, and their role was in no way threatened by the spectre of health service reorganisations.[6] As far as the role of economists who acted as advisers to the concerned government departments such as employment and the DHSS was concerned, they could afford to accept that one of the things government should do is deal humanely with a relatively small 'residuum', a phenomenon which both Stern's and Gravelle's references to 'personal characteristics' seems to imply.

The position of economists in government departments may be contrasted (as it often is by civil servants themselves) with that of sociologists. Social scientists are employed in British government are given two titles: sociologists (and graduates in psychology or any other relevant discipline working on social research) are known as 'research officers'. Economists are known as 'economic advisers'. This difference in nomenclature conceals a major difference in the influence and status of the two disciplines. Social scientists other than economists have always played a relatively marginal role in government.[7] Sociologists' and psychologists' fates depended upon that of the units they worked for. Sociologists working in government, like economists and statisticians, are regarded as resources for administrative staff. However, there is no 'Central Sociological Office' parallel to the Central Statistical Office or the Economic Advisers Office, and no centrally directed scheme of training and career development.[8] A sociologist cannot enter the civil service via the 'fast stream' directly into the grade-7 equivalent (Principal Research Officer), and will be subjected to the galling experience of seeing economists with equivalent (or fewer) qualifications begin at a higher level of seniority and remuneration. It appears that up to a point it was the sociologists or psychologists employed as 're-search officers' who saw the problem of the health of the unem-ployed as fascinating but 'not do-able'. This was not, however, a factor which differentiated them from the economists in any sharp way. It arose from one of the normal tensions involved in doing applied research: that between satisfying one's customers on the one hand and pursuing the sort of topics which might gain recognition from one's peers in the wider discipline on the other. Relationships between social disadvantage and health are of wide interest among sociologists and psychologists in the world outside Whitehall. Like all other professionals in the civil service, research officers faced in two directions – a major con-sideration in the art of policy research is to convince the cus-tomer that what he or she wants can be achieved by letting the scientists do what *they* want (Latour 1987). This is a harder task for researchers inside government than those outside. At least in principle, researchers employed in academic institutions can ap-peal to their peers (as embodied in the Research Councils) for resources to carry out work on topics of purely academic interest ('pure' as opposed to 'applied' research). On the other hand, the prizes are also great. If DHSS ministers had been persuaded to approve the sort of project proposed by PSU, this would have been a large and well funded piece of research, and the only one intended specifically to investigate the relationship between un-employment and health.

Statistics and the policy process

The third disciplinary group with which became involved in the debate were the statisticians. The first thing to be noted about the participation of members of this discipline is what 'side' they were on. British government departments employ quite a large number of professional statisticians, as they do economists and sociologists. However, no work carried out by statisticians was ever involved in the official response. This may seem surprising, especially in view of the perception of the role played by govern-ment statisticians in, for example, revisions of the unemployment figures during the latter 1980s. In the period subsequent to the unemployment and health debate it became almost a cliché to accuse government statisticians of being a mere tool of their political commanders.

The statistical work which entered the unemployment and health debate was that carried out by the team at the Social Statistics Research Unit at City University working on the LS. Although this work was carried out in an academic institution, the LS was conceived by government statisticians working for the OPCS in the early 1970s, and the data were drawn entirely from official sources: the Census, emigration and immigration records and vital returns (deaths and births). Two members of the team at City had worked at OPCS for much of their previous careers, and the nature of their involvement was influenced by the position of their disciplinary group within government. In order to understand this involvement, we need to look more closely at what was happening to government statisticians, especially those at OPCS, during the early years of the debate on unemployment and health.

The position of government statisticians is somewhere between that of economists and other social scientists. Published reports of professional meetings indicate that many senior statisticians did not consider the careers open to their colleagues in government altogether satisfactory.[9] The view has been expressed by many commentators that only government economists end up with a truly coherent occupational or career structure with ready access to the higher reaches of the civil service (Bulmer 1978, p. 37–8; Bulmer 1987, p. 16; Booth and Coates 1978; Cherns 1979, pp. 52–4). Statisticians both inside and outside of government can occasionally be heard debating the causes of the relative success of their own discipline and economics. Like the economists, they perceived two things to be important in trying to become a 'policy scientist': (a) being seen to have a firm grasp of the more abstract aspects of the appropriate discipline *first* (you have to show you *can* do 'theoretical statistics') before gaining access to policy-related work, despite what often seem to be a rather tenuous relevance of these skills in their more elaborate forms; (b) an ability to 'reconcile requirements' ('Seeing whether they want the Milk Tray or the Dairy Box') and to 'sell one's wares' to policy-makers and others.[10] Changes at OPCS subsequent to the Rayner Reviews had made some of these problems more acute, as one statistician put it:

> Before [Rayner], [OPCS] had its own money and govern-
> ment departments had to persuade it they had a project
> worth doing ... Now people look around for the best person
> to do the job. So a Department specifies ... 'This is what we
> want'. You take the cheapest purveyor of Black Magic, if
> that is your favourite flavour. That is the Rayner theory. You
> know which organisations are going to give you the Black
> Magic and which are going to give you Dairy Box, you know
> what I mean.

But there was something even more important than 'who pays' in
this account:

> people ... are really fighting battles over what their function
> is ... in general when a request comes from a Department, it
> is very, very vague, you see. So you have to formulate it
> conceptually as well as carrying it out ... That is, after all, the
> 'trad' researcher's role ... It's not really a question of paying,
> it's a question of who is really going to play the co-ordin-
> ating role, co-ordinating the outsider's ideas, the adminis-
> trators' needs, and the practicalities of doing research ...
> [But now] you tend to get economists and client depart-
> ments saying 'OPCS's job is to get what the Department
> *wants*.'

As some of the administrative civil servants pointed out, however, the professional-statistician role did not extend to relin-
quishing the less convenient aspects of one's discipline in the face
of administrative demands. For example, a statistician told me
that on one occasion while working for a health authority he had:

> proposed four measures [to be used in a resource allocation
> formula], like GHS self-reported sickness for example. It
> was quite fun. It was discussed by the Regional Team of
> Officers. Then they just chose the measure which met their
> prior intentions best. Now, if they had been Bayesians
> [laughing] ... Well, they were obviously not. They knew
> absolutely nothing about statistics. I wasn't so naive that I'd
> thought this wouldn't happen. It was the blatancy of it
> which surprised me.

He felt that part of the job of a member of his discipline was to
make clear both the underlying 'subjective and political element'
in statistical work, and also to convey to non-statisticians the
importance both of these elements and of the underlying technical
assumptions with which they might not be familiar.

During the period of the unemployment and health debate, the position of statisticians within government departments appeared to many to be becoming weaker. When discussing their part in the debate, statisticians and civil servants made frequent mention of the Rayner review of the Government Statistical Service (GSS)(see Rayner 1977, 1980, HMSO 1981). This was carried out as part of a programme of efficiency work initiated by the Civil Service Department (for an account see Metcalfe and Richards 1987, p. 115). The atmosphere in 1979–80 can be contrasted to that of the mid and late 1960s, the period of growth in employment of professional staff by government when it had been assumed that more information led to better planning. The emphasis by 1980 was on the burden to businesses of having to collect so many statistics. The review concentrated on the cost of statistics and the management of this work within individual departments: 'A customer–contractor relationship between statistics-producers and statistics-users would force each side to examine its own needs and lead to a tauter, more cost-effective service' (Metcalfe and Richard 1987, p. 118).

The review resulted in 700 recommendations and offered savings of over £19 million. Specifically, the GSS was to be cut by some 25 per cent between May 1979 and April 1984. Most of the proposals were accepted. Metcalfe and Richards point out that the notion of a 'customer' implies a 'commercial' rather than a 'professional' relationship between users and providers of services ('the customer is always right' but not the client or patient). Most notably, it led to a change in the role of the head of the GSS. Previously this role had been concentrated on issues of integrity and accuracy of statistics. Now the head of GSS was also to provide advice to top management on questions of efficiency, an additional organisational task.

The review of OPCS at first recommended cuts of only 4 per cent. This was considered quite insufficient and a further review was carried out by staff from the central Efficiency Unit, which resulted in far sharper measures. In the end OPCS did undergo a 25 per cent reduction in staff, between 1981 and 1984. The review as a whole was accompanied by an atmosphere or intense rumour and speculation:

> Given the well-developed professional network of the statisticians,[11] it was not surprising that word began to get round about what was to be proposed ... The press publicity

surrounding the review helped to spread incipient panic among statisticians and fuelled their opposition. (Metcalfe and Richards 1987, pp 121–2)

The process raised the issue of 'professional integrity' high on the agenda of debate inside and outside of Whitehall. As well as being civil servants, government statisticians have undergone specialist training which encompasses not only the transfer of skills but also of values. Accuracy and objectivity are part of their professional ideology. In addition, there is a more general notion of 'pubic service' which is common to many professions. Metcalfe and Richards comment:

members of the GSS felt the quality of statistics reflected on their professional integrity, that wider issues of the public interest were involved in the quality of statistical work undertaken and that statisticians were ultimately the only people qualified to judge this ... doubts were cast by statisticians on the possibility of attracting good new recruits to the service. (p. 127)

This was said partly because many felt they would now have to carry a burden of administrative work ('all you could get in OPCS was numerate administrators' as one commented). All this was happening at the same time as OPCS was undertaking the LS, and anxieties about recruitment were one reason why the study was taken partly outside of OPCS (see Chapter 11).

Efficiency reviews deeply affected the statisticians working inside government departments, particularly the OPCS. But these were not the only sources of discontent in the discipline. What the accounts of statisticians involved in the unemployment and health debate seem to show is a range of complaints about the relationships between themselves and other disciplinary and professional groups. These are also seen repeatedly in presidential addresses to the Royal Statistical Society and other similar published documents (see, for example, Chandler 1984, Royal Statistical Society 1968, and, for a civil service 'view', see Armstrong 1973). They include:

1. A desire to become more fully involved in the policy-making process (which led them into contact with pressure groups), but without having to abandon those aspects of their professional identity which often led to a critical and questioning stance.

2. A desire to be more involved in the substantive issues of

the research in which they participated (whether these were the effects of work on health, health inequalities, drug trials or health service planning) rather than being 'called in' merely to analyse data at a later stage in the research process (Cauliffe 1976).

3. A feeling that their discipline was being 'misused' by people who either did not understand or did not clearly state the 'underlying assumptions' involved, or the extent to which statistical 'results' themselves involve an element of choice and decision-making.

The last point was sometimes made by statisticians whom I spoke to in the form of 'Bayesian jokes'. Whenever Bayes is mentioned (which he quite often is see for example, Durbin 1987), the reference is to an alternative theory of statistics, which does not take it as a first assumption that everything in the world should be regarded as randomly distributed, but rather that the statistician explicitly begins with certain ideas about how things 'really are'. These ideas are called 'priors'. The charm of the Bayesian approach will be evident from the obvious difference it would make to any group involved in a policy-making process, as the 'priors' will have to be derived from some knowledge or understanding of the substantive issues which some statisticians wished to be credited with more often (for example see the Royal Statistical Society (RSS) evidence to the Parliamentary Estimates Committee, fourth report 1966–7, and the discussion reported in *JRSS* Series A, vol. 131, pp. 1–5). The comments made above on health authority managers reflect a tendency amongst statisticians (and perhaps other scientists in fields closely related to policy-making) to be reluctant to leave the 'priors' entirely in the hands of politicians.[12] Unfortunately, what is substantively gained by a Bayesian approach is technically lost, as the severe problems in characterising the distributions of test statistics and therefore of establishing the significance of results, have not been overcome by Bayesians.[13]

As time went on, the question of 'the integrity of government statistics' and 'Ministers ignoring expert advice' rose higher on the political agenda. For example in November 1985 Michael Meacher accused the government of a 'bunker mentality', made necessary by the fact that even 'top civil servants who do not share Ministers' poitical prejudices had been sidelined ... objective and independent advice no longer reached minister' (Travis 1985).

In the same vein, in February 1986 Jeremy Laurence wrote for *New Society* on 'How Ministers fiddle figures' (Laurence 1986), in which he enumerated the 'distortions of statistics on public spending, hypothermia deaths and the health of the unemployed'. The Central Statistical Office, he continued:

> continually finds itself in the position of having to defend its integrity ... Statistics are the bedrock of government. They supply the facts against which its politices are justified and the measure by which their success (or failure) is assessed.

A 'conspiracy theory', Laurence felt, was, in this case, not mere fantasy. Statisticians, he states in the article, fight regular battles with civil servants and ministers over the presentation of figures. Sir John Boreham, who had retired as head of the Central Statistical Office in 1985, told him; 'Governments are composed of human beings. They don't like publishing statistics that show their policies aren't working yet. That's when it gets interesting'.

According to Laurence, the statisticians felt that they 'nearly always won'. An exception had been the removal of a table on the health of the unemployed from the 1986 edition of *Social Trends*. Boreham himself had 'got as far as drafting his resignation letter once' and was aware that 'technical questions such as the recognition of hypothermia as a cause of death ... get fogged up with political questions'. Overall, however, Boreham considered that 'The government is pretty clean in this country – *because we have a bloody powerful scientific establishment*' (Laurence 1986, my emphasis, p. 362).

As time went on, it was the 'suppression of government information' which became a favourite of the media, to the extent that by 1986, most mentions of 'the effect of unemployment on health' in quality newspapers and TV documentaries were made in this connection. As *Scotsman* journalist Bryan Christie told me early in 1986, 'Death on the dole' was no longer an interesting topic for journalist: 'I wouldn't write anything more about unemployment and health now. It's quite clear that unemployment does harm health. The real story now is how civil servants are sitting on information'.

His generalisation to 'civil servants' is somewhat too broad, as the reason why journalists were becoming aware of 'suppression of information' was that some civil servants, not least government statisticians, were going as far as their situation allowed to express dissidence, in the wake of the Rayner cuts. A further twist to the spiral took place when, on 2 June 1986, yet another 'major review' of the work of OPCS was publicly announced, without warning having been given to top officials of the Office. The reaction of some officials was that the proposal to devolve some or all of the survey work of OPCS to the appropriate government departments would reduce the independence of the producers of information on social trends.

A professional boundary dispute

The combined effect of all these influences was to set up a series of potential boundary disputes between disciplinary groups within and outside of government. Macleod and Novak have documented the struggles by newly professionalising groups to claim various territories during the period of nineteenth century government growth. Knorr-Cetina has highlighted the importance of scientific entrepreneurialism in turning findings into facts. Shapin has suggested that 'professional entrepreneurialism' may provide an important link between policy processes and scientific developments. The newly felt need for appropriate knowledge within 'spending' departments had long opened up a new market into which groups could attempt to move, claiming expert status.

We have seen the importance of the role played by economists in advising government departments, and health economists were, during the period of this study swiftly establishing a more influential position in relation to health policy. Community physicians however, are marginal to medicine, and in the twentieth century, medical advisers to government have tended not to be drawn from the ranks of practising public health doctors. This rendered the relative positions of these two sub-professions more equal in the contest for intellectual hegemony over health service planning than might otherwise have been expected. Health economists can challenge the exclusive right of community physicians to the planning function in a way that, for example, physiologists and anatomists cannot threaten the hegemony of clinical specialists in hospital medicine. In particular, economic techniques such as 'satisficing' and 'sub-optimisation' fitted well into the new, increasingly managerial style of health service planning, and the implementation of the Griffiths Report strengthened the hand of the more 'managerially' oriented school of health economists still further (Ledwith 1987, St George 1985).

The conflict between the economists who claimed that unem-

ployment had little or no effect on health, and Manifesto community physicians and their academic allies from the fields of statistics and sociology was frequently couched by participants themselves in terms of the political allegiances of their opponents.
However, analysis of the progress of the debate over time seems
to point to a greater influence of professional (including 'personal
advancement') rather than political factors. Positions adopted in
relation to the 'facts' seem to have been the result of different
perceptions of potential tasks, alliances, and balances of forces
amongst the entrepreneurial and innovative members of professional and disciplinary sub-groups. The unemployment and
health debate was a field of contestation between entrepreneurial
groups within sub-professions and sub-disciplines whose aims
included both competition for a specific expert role and change
within the disciplines themselves. At issue was which profession
or discipline was successfully going to lay claim to the status of
providing appropriate expertise to those planning and administering the health service, and those charged with justifying these
policies in the eyes of the public. In order to do this, disciplinary
sub-groups sought to form alliances with professional sub-groups
('get on the bandwagon'). It would be pointless for economists to
seek allies among their 'natural competitors' in this contest, which
was what epidemiologists and medical statisticians effectively
were. The latter had long accepted (if reluctantly) a role in which
public health and other forms of medicine acted as their more
powerful client. The economists wished to go further, as one
remarked: 'After all, we can do it better than they [community
physicians] can – you don't need a medical degree to do health
service planning'.

Members of the less ambitious sub-disciplines (medical and
social statistics, medical sociology) still had to chose between
factions within the professions. There was no obvious reason why
sociologists, for example, could not have concentrated on an alliance with clinical epidemiology and community health promotion based around ideas of smoking, diet and other forms of
individual behavior and 'health beliefs' as major determinants of
population health. Business for sociologists could be generated in
the form of meticulous studies of such behaviour with putative
implications for prevention. Many did take this line, particularly
in relation to AIDS. There was nothing inevitable in the adoption
by a group within the Faculty of Community Medicine of a 'struc-

tural/environmental' model of the determinants of community health.[14] Advocates of medical audit and other forms of cost containment might well also find a use for social scientists and statisticians.

The scope for manoeuvre of the statisticians who worked on the LS was limited, however. And this was not merely because of their traditional links back to the reforming traditions of nineteeth century public health. Admittedly, it would not have seemed likely that a similar place in history to that of Chadwick could await a professional group confined to lecturing the populace on the evils of smoking and sausages. But here again 'technical interests' appear to be important. The data the LS team and other vital statisticians had to offer provided no information on behaviour or health beliefs, although the possibility of including questions on diet and smoking in the Census had been raised at a high level in OPCS. But it seems that the data they had to hand left them little choice but to ally with those within community medicine who adopted a 'structural' and environmental view of the determinants of health. This was an important addition to the long common history of involvement in influential reforming movements going back to the public health debates of the mid-nineteenth century.

Notes

1. Almost certainly a reference to the PSU.
2. For further explanation of these events see Chapter 6.
3. However, it must also be said that civil servants were critical of the factual accuracy of Prince's account of what went on during this period inside DHSS, and saw his book as more useful 'theoretically' than as a practical guide to 'what really happened' within the Department.
4. It should be pointed out that although they do not use the term, public-health oriented epidemiologists ALSO use 'production functions' ... this merely refers to the hypothesised relationship between input and output. The important difference, symbolised by different language, is in what are thought to be the biologically and politically relevant FORMS of input and outcome.
5. See, for example, Fuchs (1972) Perlman (1974), Wagstaff (1986a, 1986b).
6. The abolition of the Area tier of Health Authorities in England in 1982 had done away with some Community Physician posts, and the Griffiths proposals for General Managers threatened the position of these 'clinical managers' even more, see Ham (1986).
7. For a recent and enlightening account of the position of 'research officers' in government departments, see R. Walker (1987).

8. Though see Blume's (1987, p. 81) account of the brief life of the Social Research Co-ordinating Committee in the Cabinet Office.

9. For examples of such dissatisfaction and the continuing debate on statistical careers in government see, for example, Allen (1970), Griffin (1985)

10. Both of these may of course be seen as direct equivalents to the economists' concerns.

11. For one example of the reaction by statisticians see Hoinville and Smith 1982.

12. The absence of 'priors' in classical statistics stands in sharp contrast, of course, to the rich store of substantive 'starting points' open to economists.

13. I am grateful to Donald Mackenzie for pointing out that a sociologist of scientific knowledge should look more closely at the notion that 'Bayesian methods do not yield results whose significance can be tested', rather than unquestioningly accepting this as the reason why the approach has not been more widely used.

14. Long after the debate analysed here had died away, a young but rapidly rising advocate of the 'operational research' approach to the public health doctor's role was moved to fury by advocates of the 'structural' approach: he felt that social epidemiologists were trying to reduce practising public health doctors to the role of merely implementing policies based on the epidemiologists' research on the determinants of community health. This opposition also took the form of questioning the 'truth' of the research itself.

11

CONSTRUCTING THE SCIENTIFIC RESPONSE

The cycle of credibility

We have now seen the context within which 'the health of the unemployed' became a topic of interest to researchers. And it is at this point that a theoretical perspective which highlights the interconnections between science and policy come into its own. At the outset of this study, a guide to theory and method when considering the role played by the researchers was taken from Mackenzie's (1981a) account of the development of statistics in Britain in the early twentieth century. There were obvious reasons for this choice: Mackenzie dealt with an occupational group similar to some of the scientists in the unemployment and health issue community; a similar topic: the application of statistical methods to a politically controversial issue in public health; and used a theoretical perspective which seemed to offer a fruitful way of organising some of the material. Mackenzie was concerned with the ways in which the 'interests' derived from the social origins and class membership of the participants influenced not only the answers they gave to specific questions, but also the very methods which they used to formulate these answers, down to fine points of mathematical detail. As a result, one of the guiding ideas with which the present study began was an expectation that the social position and political allegiances of participants in the unemployment and health debate – in this case not only statisticians but also doctors, economists, and other kinds of academic and professional and paraprofessional workers – would be found to influence the stances which they took and the ways in which they went about investigating the question 'does unemployment cause ill health?' It seemed that there should have turned out to be a group of participants drawn from non-élite social groups and owing their allegiance to liberal or progressive political currents who took up, defended, and technically elaborated one position ('it does'), and another group, with élite social position or origins and conservative political allegiance, who took up and defended the opposite view.

Mackenzie's thesis to the effect that scientific developments must be understood in the context of the occupational roles open to scientific workers (see his analysis of the career of Major Greenwood, pp. 110–12) held up very strongly when used as a guide to understanding the relationship between research and policy in the unemployment debate. However, perhaps because of the different historical periods at which the two debates took place, from the beginning of the present study there were difficulties in the use of the concept of 'social interests'.

To give one example of these problems, the first few researchers who were interviewed seemed to have great difficulty in remembering what they had actually said in papers and talks about unemployment and health. Interviewed approximately eighteen months after the major Scottish conference on the subject, speakers seemed vague, almost uninterested, and told me that I must understand they had 'moved on to other things'. The topic was, to the first scientists interviewed, clearly some kind of a sideline. It obviously would not do to assume that they had carried out some work in this area either out of intellectual fascination or for (covert or explicit) 'political' reasons.

Several of them expressed considerable detachment from whatever substantive issues they might happen to find themselves working on, including the present one. Far from declaring any particular 'interest' in the question of unemployment and health, one told me: 'this sort of work is just what I happen to be doing at the moment. This is very much just a job for me'.

Another member of the same research team thought that it was very important I should understand his (as well as other peoples') work on unemployment and health as a contingent event in a normal scientific career. He gave an account of the organisation of research, and his own place within it, closely congruent with Latour and Woolgar's description of the 'cycle of credibility'.

> Do you find that a lot of people are embarrassed by making a living out of other people's lack of a living? It's a bit of a bandwagon, isn't it.? ... I was keen that [unemployment and health] shouldn't be pushed too far just because it is an OK topic and you can get money to do it. A lot of people have moved into it. A lot of people have been opportunistic in going into the field because it is an area that shows they are

doing policy-relevant work. Even if the results of the research are not going to lead to anything that's going to be
implemented ... This sort of thing happens in Medical Stats.
Fashions come and go ... It [is] easier to publish because
there [are] more people doing things like monographs and
special editions of journals. These are the sort of practical
reasons why people get into things ... you get asked to give
talks and things like that because it is of interest to a wider
group. So that you get a lot of positive reinforcement.

Despite (or perhaps because of) the clarity with which he saw the
workings of the academic cycle of credibility, this researcher had
moral and practical objections to merely being carried along by it.

This is not to suggest that some researchers' political beliefs, or
the political context of the debate had no influence upon the
progress or outcome of the debate as a whole. It is altogether
possible, and consistent with the analysis offered here, that there
could have been a different outcome if either a social democratic
or 'liberal' conservative administration had come to power at
some time during 1978–87. In Chapter 6 it is suggested that a
temporary shift in opinion within the political party in power
may have influenced the reception of one study. However, as
there is no case study such as Mackenzie's with which to compare
the present one in respect of political context, as opposed to the
social and political origins and allegiances of participants, it must
be left to future researchers to explore in detail the influence of
political context on policy-related scientific controversy. In the
unemployment and health debate, political interests were very
seldom quoted by scientists themselves as reasons for the positions they took. In addition, the social origins and broad political
allegiances of participants were characterised more by similarity
than difference. There was, therefore, a need to search more
widely for a theoretical insight which would encompass the complexity which was beginning to emerge from interview material.

Introducing some ideas from Latour and Woolgar's study of
laboratory workers seemed to be one way of dealing with the
problem. One of the earliest insights offered by the application of
their analysis to the material provided by interviews with and
observations of the researchers in the debate concerned the question of why many researchers' memories of their own work in the
field seemed rather vague. This appeared to be partly explained
by understanding that *researchers' time is an investment in the future.*

Clarification of the importance of 'time' as an investment by research workers is a valuable contribution of the laboratory studies
to the investigation of the relationship between science and
policy-making. Researchers seldom mentioned politics in relation
to their own work, though they did attribute 'political' motives to
others. In contrast the allocation of 'time' was a concern frequently expressed in interviews. Concern about the investment of
time was not confined to scientists, but was most emphasised by
this group, and was the feature which distinguished scientists'
accounts of their participation in the debate. In contrast, 'intellectual fascination' and being 'hooked' was expressed by non-
academic participants.

The different orientations to 'time' and 'moving on' of a young
academic economist and a civil servant was expressed thus in one
interview:

> Well, you see, ('x') is a civil servant, an economic adviser. So
> perhaps he goes on longer on the same subjects, because of
> their policy aspects. But for people like me [an academic
> economist], you take up a topic and then you drop it, either
> other people take it up or it fades away.

There seemed to be conflicting pressures at work. The academic
researcher's time is a part of her means of production, in the
Marxist sense: the scientist is unlike some other workers in that
she is not totally 'alienated' from the means of producing knowledge, because time is a resource over which the scientific worker
may retain some degree of 'ownership' and control. So there is
pressure for the scientist to ensure that her time is as fully in-
vested as possible (hence the negotiation of 'busy-ness' so com-
monplace in academic life.) To give a concrete example from my
own field observations, statisticians working in medical settings
set great store by being 'very busy'. Of course, they are. But also, it
was a signalling of disciplinary autonomy and professional prestige to make doctors, especially, wait in a queue for the statistician's attention. The other side of this social negotiation of 'busy-
ness' (i.e. the full investment of 'time') is, however, that some
scientists exhibited, in the present study, a tendency to over-
commit themselves at certain stages of their careers. The investment of 'time' must not only be made but must be seen to be
made. This gives rise to a tight and delicately balanced agenda of
work priorities for the scientist, in which individual items are
highly susceptible to being rescheduled to the bottom of a lengthy

list, regardless of the personal interest or commitment of the scientist. In other words, the micro-level negotiation of 'time' may, at certain points, leave little space for considerations of 'interests', whether these be overtly political or more personal commitments, perhaps derived from the scientist's social and cultural background. To be abandoned by scientists, therefore, it is not necessary that some area of investigation be 'suppressed' or 'censored'. Considerations of time management are a powerful source of control over the setting of the scientific agenda. The successful scientist will know when to terminate a poor investment, when to 'move on to other things'. The junior scientist learns this skill as part of her socialisation. Although decisions taken according to these criteria may be, at certain points, experienced as a form of 'censorship' they will normally be justifiable in terms of setting sensible work priorities, for the good of the laboratory and that of the novice's own career.

In interviews, academic scientists who had made this kind of decision in relation to 'unemployment and health' often had notable difficulties in remembering their own previous work. However, far from being a 'problem' for them (although it sometimes caused embarrassment in the interview situation, mainly due to its total incongruity with the field-worker's prior expectation),[1] this ability to 'move on' decisively was regarded as a product of experience in the proper doing of science in the real world.

Latour and Woolgar's account of the cycle of credibility and the resulting concept of academic 'time' as an investment which the experienced scientist learns to deploy artfully, allows us to perceive one of the major, if latent and unexplicated, methods of agenda-setting within science itself. What this model of scientific decision-making means is that we often have no need to look for more obvious external influences to account for the appearance or disappearance of certain questions as 'scientifically interesting' and 'worthwhile'. Because the skilful scientist will pick up far more subtle signals about 'what is hot and what is out', and follow their indications, as part of the normally competent pursuit of an academic career. This is emphatically *not* to say that politically controversial topics are written-out of science, but 'in a subtle way'. On the contrary, a topic may prove a good investment by being at a point of balance within a controversy, or may be *made into* a good investment by being strategically linked to an 'external controversy'. The entrepreneurialism involved here is also a part of successful science.

However, allocation of 'time' takes place as between activities which are by no means all defined by the scientific community itself. On the contrary, the degree to which scientists are free to pursue the goals most prized within their own professional circles can be severely limited. And at the time when Brenner's work was breaking into the British academic scene, these limitations were becoming greater.

Shifting priorities in medical research

Although 'translation theorists' such as Latour, Callon and Law lay greater emphasis on concepts of enrolment and network formation, they do not reject the concept of 'interest'.[2] But they use it in a somewhat different way to that of, for example, Barnes (1977) and Mackenzie (1981b). They regard 'interesting', or 'interessement' as a self-conscious activity of establishing a map of other participants' objectives which can be used strategically to adjust one's own.

If we look more closely at the processes which produced the three papers which appeared in 1982 and gained their authors a central place (almost what Collins would call 'core group' status) we can see how this worked in the case of unemployment and health. Two important factors need first to be understood: the ways in which attempts had been made to shift the priorities in medical research and orient them more towards 'consumer needs' than the internal criteria of disciplines; and the ways in which the application of the Rothschild principles affected social research outside government departments.

In 1971, like all other departments funding research, the DHSS appointed a Chief Scientist. The second Chief Scientist to be appointed, Sir Douglas Black, elected to play a part-time, advisory role, and worked with a 'Chief Scientist's Advisory committee' (CSRC) of experts, whose role was to assess priorities across the whole research programme. This was part of the 'Rothschild' reorganisations of government-funded research (Kogan and Henkel 1983), and on the same principle 25 per cent of the Medical Research Council's allocation from central government, which had always come from the DHSS (unlike that of other research councils which comes wholly from the DES) was transferred back to the Department to be devoted (on a contracted basis) to 'Health Services Research'. By this was meant research directed at the 'effectiveness and efficiency', appropriateness and acceptability of clinical services, especially services to the less glamorous client groups such as the mentally and physically handicapped.

Prior to the 'transfer of funds', decisions as to what research would be supported by the MRC were not taken on a 'customer–contractor' basis. The members of the Council, the key decision makers who allocated both its DES and its DHSS grants, are drawn from the 'high-tech' clinical specialities, proud of their independence and high scientific standards. As members are drawn from the clinical specialities, their priorities tended to reflect those of clinical practice and the basic medical sciences rather than those of government departments. It came as a considerable shock to find that a large chunk of their annual budget would now have to be bid for on the same customer–contractor basis as that followed by research units in government departments.

Within the DHSS in the mid-1970s, broadly, four major areas of 'R&D' may be distinguished: Health Service, Personal Social Services and Special Client Groups, NHS Equipment and Supplies, etc, and Social Security. After the transfer of funds, DHSS money also used to fund studies carried out by the MRC also appeared in the accounts. The balance sheet in the period under study looked something like Table 11.1.

From Table 11.1 can be seen the magnitude of the transferred funds from the MRC as a proportion of all research spending by the DHSS. The 'health service' topics to which these funds were intended to be devoted were a traditional area of concern to 'social medicine', and the composition of the CSRC's medical membership reflected this – the Chief Scientist, Sir Douglas Black

Table 11.1 DHSS R&D Expenditure 1976–81 (000s).

	1976/7	1977/8	1978/9	1979/80	1980/81
Health services	368	4134	4364	4865	5785
PSS/Client Grps	2594	2887	3456	4246	5326
NHS Equipmt.	2936	2614	3118	4196	5399
Soc. Security	270	329	352	353	469
MRC	8936	8920	10740	11436	13778
MRC as % of all	59.2	47.2	48.8	45.6	44.8

Source: DHSS Research and Development Handbooks
(Comparable tables were not published after 1981)

later chaired the group which produced the Black Report on Inequalities in Health (DHSS 1980). Black himself had been a leading clinical scientist, and a member of one of the MRC Research Boards. But the committee included Cochrane, Morris and another prominent figure in social medicine: Prof Alwyn Smith (an early academic participant in the UHSG). Other members during the brief life of the CSRC included social policy academics David Donnison and Peter Townsend at various points in time. Only three 'pure clinicians' (out of eighteen) were included in 1973, this rose to four (out nineteen) by 1979, the last year of the CSRC's existence.

Sir Douglas Black expressed enthusiasm at the composition of his Research Committee:

> We were lucky in the help we enlisted from outside scientists. It was a totally different set of disciplines from those [which] one thinks of in connection with clinical research; for example, sociologists, economists, statisticians and so on. It was an interesting experience, and not merely in the Chinese sense of the word. (Black 1986)

Thus the composition of the CSRC can be seen as influenced by the critique of the dominance of the clinical specialties in medicine, both in terms of intellectual hegemony and in terms of command over resources. 'clinical' dominance was regarded by many policy-makers as acting to the detriment of other services, particularly under the new conditions of economic stringency. This critique united two separate interests: the concern to limit health expenditure without arousing public protest, by discrediting that section of the medical profession which pressed for more and more resources for advanced technology, and the 'radical' rejection of mechanistic forms of medicine, which originated outside of government. During its short existence, the Chief Scientist's Research Committee of the DHSS expressed the claims of social medicine and public health to set new priorities for health research.

In Black's view, it was the restrictions on resources and civil service staffing that resulted from organisational reviews which hindered the ability of the DHSS to continue administering the transferred MRC funds on a 'Rothschild' basis. Additionally, however, as also discussed by Kogan and Henkel, there was the inherent conflict between politically determined priorities (in this case, services to the 'priority client groups' of older people and people with disabilities) and what Black termed 'the question of scientific opportunity'. In other words, how to strike the balance between unglamorous, service-oriented research on the elderly, disability and problems of service delivery and those topics which 'good' scientists wished to pursue in order to gain prestige in the eyes of peers? This was made even more difficult by the fact that even in the case of service-oriented research, it was not easy to 'identify a customer'. According to Black, the most likely candidate was:

> An Under-Secretary in charge of 18 or 19 Divisions in the DHSS ... They vary in their devotion to the furthering of research, and given that research is only about 1 per cent of their total budget, this is only natural ... Bureaucracy arose from the necessity to identify a credible customer.

And a civil service research manager remarked, 'the CSRC ... was supposed to be an overarching research strategy committee. But the Departments just don't *have* strategies'.

In 1978, Sir Arthur Buller took over as full time chief scientist and the CSRC was dismantled.[3] In 1979 all DHSS funded research units began to be reviewed with a view to cut-backs. At the same time, the MRC's role was once again recovering strength. In 1981, the funds transferred to the DHSS were handed back, on the condition that the MRC undertake to fund more research decided on the basis of 'need' and policy relevance rather than judgements of scientific merit alone. In order to facilitate this, a Health Services Research Panel was set up within the MRC, which included members from the DHSS and Department of Employment. This arrangement was termed the 'Concordat'.

Analysing the researchers' involvement

The combined effect of all these changes was to create a situation where the MRC, although once more in control of the 'transferred 25 per cent' of funds, had become more sensitive to the priorities of government departments. At the same time, the traditional divisions between departmental concerns made it difficult to respond to an issue which so clearly crossed departmental boundaries. It is not surprising therefore to see that government departments were limited in the opposing claims they could make to those of the supporters of Brenner. A quick beginning to the 'official response' phase of the debate was provided by the work work of two DHSS economic advisers, Ramsden and Smee, and

by three other economists with links to government (one had
worked in the DHSS and on of the others had acted as an adviser
on health policy questions). But a space was opened up by the
combination of circumstances: the media were unsure whether to
regard the question as 'settled'; the pressure groups were down
but not out after Gravelle *et al.*'s paper in late 1981. On the other
hand, the Concordat had heightened the awareness of research
teams funded by the MRC to the demand for 'policy-relevant
work'. This produced an opportunity for some entrepreneurialism by senior academics, aware of the obligation of the MRC
under the Concordat to look more favourably on 'unmarried
mother type problems', and hoping that government as well as
MRC funding could be a little more likely to be forthcoming in
view of the political impact of Brenner's work. It was common
knowledge that the Health Services Research Panel of the MRC
was having trouble finding enough projects to fund which fitted
both the criteria of policy or service relevance and 'scientific respectability'. As one civil servant saw it, '[unemployment and
health] was a good political customer-potential exercise desper-
ately in search of a hypothesis. People felt "Here is a good subject
that we can get money on!" It was a bandwagon'.

This does not means that the research teams who produced the
three pieces of work which entered the debate in 1982 and influenced its progress decided to take up 'unemployment and health'
in a deliberately calculating manner. This would be as great a
distortion as regarding their actions as motivated by 'political or
social interests'. Rather, the Concordat and the travails of the
MRC's Health Services Research Panel may be regarded as part of
the 'interest map' of researchers, just as their own political, social
and intellectual commitments were.

There were three existing research programmes with some
track record in the area of the relationship between health and
social conditions who produced information that was fed into the
unemployment and health debate. We can understand their contribution in terms of these programmes' relationship to previous
social-problem debates. Interests and enrolment processes which
had influenced directions of inquiry in the distant past can be
seen to have left their traces on whole research programmes.
These then shaped the possibilities and limitations of the answers
which teams of researchers could offer to the question 'does
unemployment harm health?' The research programmes will be

discussed in the order in which their first published work on unemployment and health appeared.

The British Regional Heart Study (BRHS)

The initial impetus for the setting-up of this major prospective study of the causes of coronary heart disease might appear far removed from unemployment. The rationale for the initial MRC grant in 1975, was the investigation of the relationship between heart disease and hardness of water supplies. And yet, the history of the MRC Social Medicine Unit, from where the research originated, tells a different story.

In 1948, one author of the pioneer epidemiological paper on health and recession (Morris and Titmuss 1944), J. N. Morris, was appointed Director of a new MRC Social Medicine Research Unit at the Central Middlesex Hospital. Early projects included the investigation of the occupational incidence of heart disease in middle life (Committee of the Privy Council for Medical Research, 1949, p. 180). An early member of the staff was Richard Titmuss, co-author of the 1944 paper.[4]

In the academic year 1955–6, the unit's staff was joined by Dr M. D. Crawford. In 1961, she published, in association with Morris and J. A. Heady, who in that year became Assistant Director of the unit, a paper on 'Hardness of water supplies and mortality from cardiovascular disease in the county boroughs of England and Wales' (Crawford, Morris and Heady 1961). In 1962 Peter Draper joined the Social Medicine Unit, and stayed until November 1964. During this period the basic research programme included work on juvenile delinquency, mental illness and pollution of air and water, but heart disease seems to become a more dominant concern. On 30 September 1967 Morris was appointed to the Chair of Public Health at the London School of Hygiene and Tropical Medicine (LSHTM),[5] and the Social Medicine Unit moved with him. It seems that Crawford's work on water hardness was the most successful aspect of the unit's work at this time. In the School's annual report for 1968–9 (LSHTM, 1969) some prominence is given to it, and to an account of further work planned on mortality in twelve soft water and twelve hard-water towns. This was the sort of work which 'social medicine' had envisaged and, in addition, it aimed to overcome some traditional antipathies[6] by being undertaken in collaboration with the local Medical Officers of Health.

In January 1970, Dr A. G. Shaper, who had previously been Research Professor in Cardiovascular Diseases at Makerere University College, joined the staff of the unit. The MRC's annual reports from 1971–2 onwards betray new concerns following on the implementation of the Rothschild reforms. It does appear that concern with 'arterial disease' and the causes of the kind of change and damage in blood vessels which is thought to eventuate in heart attacks was seen as a topic which would appeal both to scientists and to 'customers' in government. In the words of member of the British Regional Heart Study staff, it seemed that this might pose a 'classic public health problem' – that is, water quality might turn out to be the sort of aetiological factor which could only be affected by 'mass intervention' of a type which would have to be sanctioned by government (the most successful example of this was perhaps the Clean Air Acts; another example of such an issue would be water fluoridation to prevent tooth decay.) It also involved combining epidemiological skills with the more traditionally, highly-valued clinical skills which were needed to frame hypotheses about the possible pathways by which water constituents might affect the heart, and to integrate the results of case histories, blood chemistry, electrocardiography, spirometry, etc.

In 1975, the Social Medicine Unit was wound up, on the retirement of Morris. As funds had been obtained from the MRC for the Regional Heart Study in the form of a five year 'Programme Grant', Shaper, who became study director, moved, project and all, to the medical school at the Royal Free Hospital, where he took up the chair of clinical epidemiology. The design of the Regional Heart Study reflected aspects of the method adopted by Morris and Titmuss in the 1930s (Morris and Titmuss 1944, see also discussion by Bartley 1987), and continued by the work on regional variations in mortality begun by Morris, Crawford and Gardner at the Social Medicine Unit. Its purpose was to investigate a possible link between heart disease and softness of drinking water. Accordingly the study's twenty-four towns were chosen to represent all combinations of water quality and heart disease mortality – so that investigation could be made into the 'exceptions': those towns with high heart disease and hard water and vice versa. As well as ECG and blood pressure and blood lipid tests, the water in the homes of 10 per cent of the men examined was analysed by the Water Research Centre at Henley.

At the beginning of the academic year 1980–81, the team was joined by an American Millbank scholar, doing the practical work for an MSc in Epidemiology at the London School of Hygiene, Richard Cummins. Cummins was from Arkansas, had graduated from the progressively-inclined Case Western Reserve medical school, and worked in programmes designed to bring medical care to under-served poverty areas. During his period on the Regional Heart Study he did some work on smoking and drinking behaviour, and in the process teamed up with a GP who was doing some 'sessional' teaching in the Department, Ray Hume. Hume was interested in tranquilliser use, in particular the idea that if patients were withdrawn too quickly from tranquillisers, they might turn to alcohol. Running through the data, they discovered that an unexpectedly large number (in view of their age and gender) of the study's subjects were taking tranquillisers. It also appeared that one factor significantly associated with tranquilliser use was unemployment. As a more or less accidental product of the coding of occupations, 408 men were found to be unemployed, most of them (according to their own accounts) 'because of ill health'.

Also quite by chance, a medical sociologist was employed in the department at this time as a technical assistant. Cummins and Hume approached her, assuming that sociologists would know about unemployment. The sociologist in fact knew nothing about unemployment (not a topic for undergratuate sociology courses during her college days) but had met Adrian Sinfield while working at Essex some fifteen years previously. At around this time, Sinfield's book *What Unemployment Means* had been published, and she had seen him interviewed on television about it. The book, hastily borrowed from a local public library, offered some ideas on how to proceed. The ideas, in turn, offered a possibility to collaborate in a paper on a topic which had suddenly become 'hot' in epidemiology.

At this stage, Hume and Cummins also enlisted the help of one of the statisticians working on the study, Derek Cook, to do some more complex analysis of their results, and also of the study director Gerry Shaper. The results of running employment status against health variables, at first sight, were quite striking. Even after making allowances for the fact that a high proportion of men said that their health was the reason for their unemployment, the group decided their paper was worth publication, in view of the topicality of the subject. It was the first paper from the Regional Heart Study to appear in *The Lancet*.

The OPCS LS

On 9 June 1982, three days after the BRHS paper, the monograph *Socio-Demographic Differentials in Mortality* appeared, published by Her Majesty's Stationary Office. It was press-released and provoked more media response than that by Cook and colleagues, for example a *Times* piece on page 2 headed 'Unemployed have higher death rate – study shows' by Nicholas Timmins. It reported that the results showed a death rate from accidents and violent causes, including suicide, amongst the unemployed well over twice as high as that for men in work, and a death rate from cancer half again as high as that for the employed.[7]

The origins of the LS lay in two domains: professional and official. From the professional domain there were the same 'technical interests' discussed in Chapter 8, the feeling that new techniques both of data handling and analysis could be used to increase understanding of population trends. From the official domain had emerged, in the early 1970s, a suspicion that existing routine statistics were tending to exaggerate class differences in mortality.

Traditionally, measures of mortality differences between occupations and social classes are given by The Registrar-General's *Decennial Supplements* (DS) which accompany (usually at considerable delay) each Census. To get mortality rates in different social classes the denominator (i.e. the numbers in each social class) is derived from the census count. The numerator (the number of deaths occurring to members of each social class, usually in a three-year period around the Census date) is taken from the occupations stated on death certificates. There is a problem arising from the use of different sources to establish the numerator and the denominator. As discussed by various commentators (Leete and Fox 1977; OPCS 1986 pp. 12–17) this gives rise to the risk of 'ecological fallacy' and 'numerator-denominator bias'. Who is to say that those who die in a certain social class have spent most of their lives there? Could lower classes have higher mortality because the sick are downwardly mobile into these classes? These were some of the questions the LS was set up to answer (see the discussion in OPCS 1973). It was to do so by following *the same individuals* from (eventually) birth to death.

According to a senior government research manager, the first initiative which led to the setting up of the LS 'came from the General Register Office' because of concern about the comparability of information about social class obtained at death registration and at Census.

> It is the business of this office to produce classifications which are meaningful and useful, and concepts of what is meaningful and useful change ... The specific debate in 1973 was) the validity of the [social-class-specific] mortality rates ... Our story was ... traditionally we have produced social class differentials [in mortality and fertility rates] so we could say that we could do our job better with a longitudinal study.

The idea of a longitudinal study of one per cent of the population had also been linked to moves towards quinquennial Censuses, and a growing interest in 'record linkage' as in aid to population surveillance and planning.[8] So, in the early 1970s, it had been thought that there would be a *five*-yearly input into the LS, which would have allowed access to much greater detail on the succession of events occurring to sample members. As one administrator put it: 'In the early 1970s, you see, planning was all the rage, and we felt that planning purposes required more frequent Censuses'. The task of following one per cent of the 1971 population, linking Census records to records of births, deaths and cancer registration, and then on to 1981 data, did prove formidable. It was not until 1975 that the one per cent sample of the 1971 Census had even been assembled, and no reports appeared until 1979.

In 1975 John Fox had been recruited from the Health and Safety Executive to write the Decennial Supplement on Occupational Mortality to the 1971 Census. While still working on the DS (OPCS 1978), Fox became interested in the idea of the LS and began to assemble some resources to push the analysis forward. In 1979, he argued that a team of full-time personnel would be needed. Many at OPCS agreed with this, but at the time of restraint on civil-service recruitment, there would have been little chance of staff being allocated to the study. So Fox decided to apply for a two-year Professorial Research Fellowship in the Department of Mathematics at City University, and asked OPCS if he could try and obtain outside funding to build up a research team. He obtained funds, eventually, from the Cancer Research Campaign (for a post which was taken up in 1980) and the SSRC (as it was then) in 1981. The OPCS continued to cover the costs of half Fox's salary and the heavy costs of data processing. These were the resources which lay behind the production of the first monograph. As a result, the team working on the LS felt all the same pressures of other contract researchers – the study must be made to demonstrate its worth by tackling subjects which would attract interest and funding from a variety of organisations.

The LS sample was drawn by choosing four days in the year and including anyone born on that day (because 4/364 = approximately 1 per cent). In all subsequent years, new births or immigrations taking place on any of those four dates were added to the sample. In principle, data on each individual from each Census would be added. This meant that occupation and economic position would only be available every ten years. The study could really only claim, therefore, to measure long-term changes in occupational status or employment status, and was unsuitable as an indicator of short-term mobility within, and in and out of, the labour market.

As early as 1979, Fox had published a paper in the *Annals of Occupational Hygiene* which included a table showing raised mortality amongst those classified as 'seeking work' in the week before the 1971 Census (Fox 1979). The paper went totally unremarked except by workers on the DHSS CS who were preparing the third-interview phase of their survey, and had decided to include a question on health, in order to make the CS's results relevant to policy-makers disturbed by *The Reckoning*. Prior to this time, contact between the two studies' personnel had, perhaps surprisingly, been low though one government statistician remarked that back in 1978 a DHSS scientific adviser had 'offered the Cohort Study to OPCS and some idiot turned it down'.

However, political events had changed attitudes temporarily (contact between the two studies did not last very long). There are two accounts of what happened next in my field notes: one given on a formal occasion (a presentation of results at an ESRC funded seminar on Employment and Unemployment) and the other informally. According to the formal account, 'The Department of Employment and the DHSS approached us [the LS team] to see if we were interested in doing research on unemployment and health. However, in the end we went to the MRC, and other bodies, for our funding.' According to the 'informal' account, a professional adviser at the Department of Employment had suggested 'over lunch' that they take another look at the data first presented in the *Annals of Occupational Hygiene* paper. Although this account displays the importance of informal networks, in this case the LS researchers decided not to proceed on the basis of mere social contact. They asked that the Department of Employment officially approach the Registrar General and make the request in writing; this never happened. The Department of Employment never funded any work on the LS, and the DHSS did not do so until late 1985. Like their colleagues in the BRHS and in Edinburgh, the LS researchers turned their attention to unemployment and health in the normal course of their MRC funded programme, as Fox explained on 26 October 1984 (see Chapter 6) in answer to a challenge from Brenner.

They initially found that by 1976 the SMR for men of working age who reported themselves to be 'seeking work' on Census night 1971 was 130, that is, their age-standardised death rate was 30 per cent above that for all men. Fox and Goldblatt noted that 'there are no clear health grounds for expecting this category to record high mortality' (Fox and Goldblatt 1982, p. 26) and suggest that it may be an effect of the social class distribution of the unemployed, i.e. the tendency for unemployment to be concentrated in the lower and less healthy classes. This point was easily dealt with by adjusting for social class and finding that an excess still remained. This was also done when deaths for the whole period 1971–81 became available (see Chapter 5), with similar results. The excess could also be due to the higher risk of losing a job experienced by men who are already ill. Or there could be some effect of unemployment on the risk of mortality.

How could the choice be made between these last two types of explanation? As we have already seen, it was widely agreed that a longitudinal study would be needed to 'settle the question'. During 1982 and early 1983 a design for such a study was indeed under consideration by government departments, who decided against it. LS staff when interviewed made no mention of any knowledge of this. They were faced with the question of 'causation versus selection' in the same way as anyone in their disciplines would be. The problem was that the censuses of 1971 and 1981, from which LS information is drawn, contain no questions on state of health. It was therefore impossible to see whether men seeking work on census night were in any better or worse health than anyone else. Or was it?

At this point, the LS researchers took an important step, which depended on the validity of an analogy between two different types of epidemiological work: occupational health studies and studies of general populations. In studies of suspected occupational hazards, account has to be taken of what is known as the 'healthy worker effect'. By this is meant the consistent finding that mortality rates for men with *any* kind of work are lower than general population age-specific rates, which include those not in the workforce at all (this effect is far stronger in women). If followed over time, however, it can be seen that these low mortality rates return back to the level for the population as a whole, that is, in the jargon, the healthy worker effect 'wears off'.[9] It is therefore considered necessary to choose, as a control group in studies of possible industrial hazards, not a sample of the general population, but a sample from another industry which may be regarded as similarly selected for good health. Otherwise, the healthy worker effect may conceal the effect of the hazard.

The 'healthy worker' effect is duly observed in the LS sample, with, between 1971 and 1975, the 3021 deaths of men employed on Census night 1971 giving an SMR (ratio of observed deaths to those expected if the death rate of the employed had been the same as that for 'all men' – i.e. employed, unemployed, retired, permanently and temporarily sick, and students) of only eighty-six. The healthy worker effect was so strong that in the first five years following the 1971 Census, all members of the LS sample allocated to any occupation experienced low mortality rates. In addition, mortality in that group of men who reported at census that they were (in the works of the census schedule) 'seeking work' began at a relatively low level. The excess only appeared after more than two years of follow up.

What was important for the unemployment and health debate was to be the use made by Fox and his colleagues of the way in which mortality rates varied over time, and the way in which this pattern differed between the 'seeking work' and the 'unoccupied/permanently sick'. They argued that their data showed that workers out of the labour force for reasons of long term illness (which the census does record) have very high mortality from the beginning of follow-up. But this high level also shows a tendency to 'wear off' over time. So the pattern of mortality in the permanently sick was in fact the opposite to that in the 'actively seeking work'. Whatever produced the high mortality in the 'unemployed-seeking work' was, therefore, not the same as that (pre-existing illness) which did so in the 'permanent sick'. As we have seen in Part I, their interpretation of what their data could show about the effect of unemployment on health hung crucially upon this argument.

The work of the MRC Unit for Epidemiological Studies in Psychiatry

Of those three studies which most influenced the debate after 1982, the one whose results were reported last of all was probably the one which had the greatest media impact. Like the other two, it was carried out by full-time researchers funded by the independent MRC (though not funded explicitly to do research on unemployment and health). The authors were two members of the MRC's Scientific Staff in a long-established research unit in Edinburgh. It will be worthwhile, in this case also, to give an account of the development of the Unit's work, which provides an example of the way in which another scientific team become involved in 'social problem claims-making'.

The Unit began to operate in April of 1960 in London, directed by a psychiatrist, Prof G. M. Carstairs. In January 1961, Carstairs was appointed to the Chair of Psychological Medicine at Edinburgh University and, as is the custom with MRC Units, this one moved (in April 1961) with its Director. The interests of Carstairs did not include unemployment as a specific topic. However, the unit's ethos partook of the rationalist and optimistic spirit of the time in regard to health planning:

> Epidemiological studies have two principal purposes [said an early Unit progress report]. The first is to explore aetiological factors in mental illness; the second is to estimate needs and evaluate treatment services ... the former will in the long run provide information enabling prevention and treatment to become rational instead of empirical. (*Unit Progress Report for 1960–64*, 21 May 1964, p. 1)

From the start, the Unit formed a link with the Edinburgh Regional Poisoning Treatment Centre (RPTC), at this time a ward (Ward III) of the Royal Infirmary, which received over 90 per cent of all cases of self-poisoning and self-injury in the city that required hospitalisation. The first study of the aetiology of what was later to become known as parasuicide (the phrase 'attempted suicide' was still in use at this time) explored the clinical, social, demographic and ecological characteristics of cases – this included social class but not employment status. There seems to have been a plan at this time to set up RPTCs in all major British cities.

The 'social problem' of parasuicide continued to grow. Rates of parasuicide amongst young men had trebled between 1962 and 1967. In 1968 a PhD student, Alex Robertson, had joined the Unit to undertake a study of young working class male parasuicides (*Unit Progress Report*, October 1974, p. 7). It seemed that these young men had been subjected to a particularly high frequency of life events.

Dr Norman Kreitman joined the Unit's scientific staff in January 1966, and became Director in April 1971. By this time, studies of suicide and 'attempted suicide' took a prominent place in the Unit's work. Parasuicide was seen as being 'on the increase' and was found to be correlated with overcrowding, juvenile delinquency, divorce, and residence in tenement dwellings. By November of 1971, studies of completed suicide and parasuicide had become the Unit's major research activity. One hypothesis now being explored was that certain 'problem' areas with high parasuicide rates were characterised by a 'subculture of parasuicide' in which self-destructive behaviour was regarded as normal or acceptable (*Unit Progress Report*, November 1971, p. 3). Stephen Platt joined the Unit in June of 1977, and started work on the 'subculture' theory for his PhD (supervised by Alex Robertson).

In the period 1977–9 rates of parasuicide had been falling by 10 per cent annually. This trend puzzled Unit staff, as 'the changes [among males] were largely due to fewer short-term re-admissions and a decrease in "acute situational reaction" presentations, despite increasing economic recession and unemployment in the community.' They seem to have been unaware of a temporary fall in the rate of unemployment during 1977 to late 1979. The Unit's progress report for 1978–81 admits that if a choice were to be forced upon it, studies of suicidal behaviour would have to be placed fourth (and last) in its order of research priorities. But by June 1981, the Unit was beginning to suffer from a contraction in research funding. Only one project on suicide remained. The priority in research was now alcohol and alcoholism.

During 1981, Norman Kreitman had come under some pressure from the MRC to develop work on unemployment in the Unit, but no definite plans were made, as few staff had any interest or expertise in the area. However, as part of his work on

parasuicide, Platt had been using data from the Regional Poisoning Treatment Centre. When discussions about unemployment
resulted from the 1981 review of the Unit's finance by an MRC
subcommittee, he remembered that data collected on each admis-
sion included employment status. At around this time a member
of the UHSG, Gill Westcott wrote to the Unit asking if anyone
there would be willing to give a paper on unemployment and
suicidal behavior at a World Health Organisation conference to be
held in Leeds in December 1982. 'That' Platt recalled 'gave me a
deadline'. As he looked at the possibilities of the RPTC data he
became increasingly excited by them. He thought that they could
both throw new light on structural factors in parasuicide and, in
more abstract methodological terms, provide an opportunity to
carry out an epidemiological exercise combining individual and
aggregate levels of analysis.

Like John Fox, Steve Platt transferred a set of ideas from
previous work into his work on unemployment and suicideal
behaviour. Fox and his colleagues at the Health and Safety Executive in the early 1970s had been suspicious of the low mortality in
workers exposed to a variety of hazards (Fox and Collier 1976).
They had used the notion of the 'healthy worker effect' to correct
for the possible distortion introduced into studies of industrial
health by the fact that employers select as their employees a
relatively 'healthy' group of people in the first place. Whereas Fox
carried over the model of the healthy worker effect by analogy,
Platt was attracted to using unemployment as a 'structural' variable in the study of parasuicide precisely because it was so different from the 'cultural' factors involved in his PhD. (Platt 1984, pp.
74–5). For some time he had been worried about the potential
misuse of research using any 'subcultural' theory of social phenomena. The work of Henderson (in, for example, Henderson and
Williams 1974) seemed to him to suggest potentially that
parasuicide should be 're-criminalised' in order to combat it, and
had gained, Platt felt, unjustifiably wide currency and credibility
both in academic and policy circles. He remembered the ways in
which the work of Oscar Lewis (who also wrote about Latin
American society) had been 'misused' in the 'culture of poverty'
debate in the United States to justify neglect of the problems of the
urban poor, and to distract attention from 'structural' causes of
poverty.

The paper reporting Platt's first findings derived from studying

the associations between parasuicide and unemployment was
published in the *Unemployment Unit Bulletin* in November 1982
(Platt 1982). The paper made no claims that unemployment necessarily exerted a 'causal' effect on suicide. It was a cautious account
of his research to date, very much in the model of MRC-funded
work, despite the somewhat unorthodox nature of the journal. *The
Unemployment Unit*, like the MRC (and notwithstanding its status
as a 'intermediate body' with the reputation of being 'political')
placed high value on balance and impartiality, which it maintained despite its explicitly campaigning purpose. Platt concluded:

> My own view is that the weight of evidence provides some
> ground for suggesting that the risk of both unemployment
> and suicide are elevated by the presence of psychiatric ill-
> ness (especially depression), rather than that unemploy-
> ment is an immediate cause of suicide. This is not to deny,
> however, that joblessness may indeed constitute an impor-
> tant intervening or moderator variable affecting the strength
> of the association between psychiatric illness and suicide.
> (Platt 1982, p. 5)

This work on suicide laid the foundations for the analysis of the
RPTC figures on parasuicide amongst the unemployed, which
came to public attention during 1983. It claims no more than that
unemployment is an 'intervening' or 'exacerbating' factor which
comes between personal states and characteristics and suicidal
behavior. As later described in the Unit's Report to the Medical
Research Council for the quinquennium 1981–86:

> At an individual level the rates of parasuicide among the
> unemployed have declined, suggesting a progressive dilu-
> tion of the pool of the unemployed with respect to personal
> pathologies. The relative risk for parasuicide of being unem-
> ployed varies according to how dominant unemployment is
> in various … subgroups.

This synopsis demonstrates the disadvantages of presenting
results with the degree of caution and impartiality valued in
scientific orthodoxy. Platt was 'playing the game according to the
rules'. He made no claim to disprove the possibility that suicidal
behaviour might arise in part from personal psychological
tendencies in unemployed people. This interpretation was later to
hinder attempts to present the effect of unemployment on self-
destructive behaviour as a 'public health problem' rather than an
individual one.

We can see from the account presented in this chapter of the origins of the three studies which provided the most important data used in the rest of the debate that adoption of 'the health of the unemployed' as a social problem worthy of research was a move which emerged out of the research teams' previous participation in debates on quite different types of social/medical 'problems'. A role was also played by the growing pressure on scientific research groups to take up policy-relevant topics at a time of shrinking resources. Senior researchers' perceived a need for the work of their 'laboratories' to appear 'policy-relevant' and 'service oriented' in the light of the extension of the Rothschild principles into medical and social research. Restrictions on funding also made the 'normal' types of scientific entrepreneurialism all the more important.

But we can also see that within this context, characteristics of the normal career or 'cycle of credibility' of scientists played an important role. As also did 'mere chance' the presence of 'socially-minded' individuals in research teams, the phone call from the media, the Director's holiday, the lunch with someone from another government department. However, the sparks of chance then fell upon a tinder of professional interests, institutional change and conflict, and wider social trends. In 1982, the ethos of MRC research groups was not compatible with a conscious search for media attention ('soap box methods'). In fact it is ironic that the one study given a press release was the one which used 'official' government figures, the LS; this is a routine practice. Young researchers such as Cook and Platt were hesitant about seeking public attention for their work – early results of the BRHS were tactfully concealed from interested inquiries by members of the British Society for Social Responsiblity in Science's 'Hazards Bulletin' for example. Contraction of funding has since then changed the policy of the MRC and other research councils towards a concern with 'dissemination'. But in the early 1980s the low profile of the studies, and the tendency towards an impartial presentation giving weight to alternative interpretations of data, which led to some disappointment for the researchers, was considered a proper form of presentation for 'real science'.

Notes

1. Qualitative data 'kicking back' again.
2. Shapin (1988) points out that although Latour appears to reject the notion of 'interest', it is in fact still strongly present in his

work, if 'smuggled through the backdoor'.

3. For an account of this see Ashworth 1984, p. 32.

4. On Titmuss' death in 1973, the annual report of the council went so far as to state, in his obituary, that working as Deputy Director of the Social Medicine Unit 'provided the stepping stone to his academic career' (MRC 1974, p. 153).

5. He was Major Greenwood's successor.

6. As discussed in Chapter 9.

7. It should be noted here that the article in *The Times* more or less allows readers to define for themselves what is meant by 'the unemployed'. In fact, 'unemployment' in this study is operationalised as 'seeking work' in the week before Census night 1971'

8. See Acheson 1967, 1968; Dr Donald Acheson later became Chief Medical Officer at the DHSS and chaired the committee on the future of communy medicine and the public health function set up in 1986. In 1966 a 10 per cent Census was carried out, and plans for a 1976 Census were only cancelled at the last moment (Whitehead 1984).

9. For a clear explanation of this idea, see Carpenter 1987.

12

UNRAVELLING THE NETWORK

In Chapter 11 we have seen something of the 'interest maps' within which those who did original research on the health of the unemployed were located. We have traced some of the alliances they made and the enrolment processes in which they were involved. The emergence of mass unemployment as a social problem, and its adoption by a 'social medicine' oriented faction within public health medicine combined with changes in the organisation of research funding to reactivate latent concerns with public health built into the research programmes themselves. Such processes are not, however, sufficient to produce 'facts'. According to the translation model, in order to become accepted as fact, knowledge claims need to become 'points of passage'. That is, they must attract the assent of a network of groups all of which see a way to their disparate goals which involves acceptance of a statement (fact') or use of an artefact which embodies the knowledge claim (the thermometer is a good example of the latter). Before this can happen the statement (or machine) must be picked up and passed on intact beyond it originators to a wider audience.

Chapters 9, 10 and 11 have analysed the forces bringing an actor-network together around the claim that unemployment causes ill health and mortality, describing the reasons why the various groups become 'interested' in the topic. As I have interpreted the story, a key concept which formed a potential obligatory point of passage was the notion of the 'wearing off of selection'. In theory, the excess morbidity in unemployed men in the BRHS and the excess suicidal behaviour found in Platt's unemployed could have indicated that unemployed men were already ill (physically or mentally). If this were true then a selective mechanism would be producing the excess mortality in the LS. But the LS researchers argued that if excess mortality in any group were produced in this way, once all members who were already 'ill' had died, the excess should disappear. That is, once the ill people had died, producing high mortality in the shorter term, the level in the group (say, the unemployed) should disappear. Unemployment itself would then be shown to have no independent effect. As this 'wearing off' pattern was not found among the unemployed in the LS, it could be argued that unemployment was exerting some causal effect – even healthy people made unemployed experienced higher risks.

Those researchers who advanced this idea did not do so initially to support a claim about the health of the unemployed. It was first used in relation to more general question of health inequalities between social groups (Fox and Goldblatt 1982, Bartley 1990). It might have had the effect of enrolling groups beyond the issue community concerned with unemployment and health – the 'poverty lobby' for example. The concept of the 'wearing off of selection' was a method of distinguishing between group-specific patterns of mortality which could be attributed to pre-existing states such as physical 'unfitness', psychological vulnerability and even habits such as smoking and drinking, from those which could not. The present author has speculated elsewhere (Bartley 1985) that after Richard Titmuss left Morris's Social Medicine Unit to take up the Chair of Social Policy at the LSE 'social policy and social medicine took separate roads'. At some points in the unemployment and health debate these roads appeared tentatively to converge once again. A better understanding of the social processes underlying the figures yielded by the LS might have been approached using ideas on social structure and social policy developed on the 'other' road, and exemplified in work such as that of Sinfield (1981), Daniel (1983) and White (1983). At the more general level of arguments about health inequalities, one always had the impression that Titmuss himself would not have been at all surprised by all this. He and Morris had written of the serious consequences for health of unemployment in the 1930s (Morris and Titmuss 1944). Furthermore, Titmuss wrote extensively of the continuation of social and economic inequality in the post-war 'welfare state', a term he never used without quotation marks. The growth of what he termed 'occupational welfare', and the other ways in which the 'welfare state' was of greater benefit to the middle classes would have made perfect sense of apparently puzzling trends such as a slight widening in social class differences in mortality, and a possible increase in the relative deprivations involved in loss of employment as the post-war years passed.

But we have also seen the end of the story (Chapter 7). When a major paper from the LS team on the health of men seeking work in the week of the 1981 Census was published in January of 1987, it received no publicity at all and had no impact on future debates about policy relating to the unemployed. The LS team was disbanded shortly afterwards. Their ideas do not seem to have disseminated beyond disciplinary barriers.

In order to understand how this happened, we need to see the ways in which those actor networks which give ideas their circulation are constantly formed, re-formed and dispersed. The network which produced accounts of unemployment's effect on mental and physical health as a social problem listed as its major participants medical statisticians and sociologists doing research in academic institutions and policy researchers in government departments. But the issue was created as an important concern by other groups, spearheaded by representatives of the 'Manifesto' tendency in community medicine and including enthusiasts for the 'community development' approach to health education, and new paraprofessions such health promotion and community psychiatry, all of which were represented at one time or another in the attendance at UHSG and Social Costs of Unemployment meetings and at the Leeds workshop in 1983. As well as their professional interests, some of these same individuals aimed to influence Labour party policy on both health and employment. As long as all of these saw a point in participating in the process of fact-building, they remained allies, even if distant ones, to the researchers who suspected unemployment damaged health.

It was not the defeat of the researchers' factual claims which broke the network, on the contrary. As Latour (1987) has it:

> There is something still worse ... than being criticised ... it is being *ignored* ... you may have written a paper that settles a fierce controversy once and for all, but if readers ignore it it cannot be turned into a fact ... Fact construction is so much a collective process that an isolated person builds only a dream. (pp. 40–1)
>
> A statement is ... always in jeopardy, much like the ball in a game of rugby. If no player takes it up it simply sits on the grass ... The total movement of ... a statement ... will depend to some extent on [the scientists'] action but to a much

greater extent on that of a crowd over which [the scientists] have little control. (p. 104)

What seems to have happened is that the actor-network which made use of the notion that unemployment harmed health left the scientists behind either because new directions opened up for them, or because the statement was well enough accepted for their purposes. The other groups in the network no longer had need of the scientists' more sophisticated constructions such as the 'wearing-off of selection' to help them achieve the purposes they aimed for. The legitimacy of 'alleviation' measures no longer required yet more sophisticated technical arguments to support it. A comparison can be made here with new drugs in medicine. Once a drug is accepted by the relevant network of prescribers and consumer (becomes a 'black box'), it little matters if neither of these groups understands the chemistry and biology involved. The whole system of side-effect notification acknowledges that there is always an element of trust involved in this, and there are not infrequent discoveries that accepted drugs can be useless or even dangerous. It should not therefore be assumed that the fragility of new knowledge is anything unique to the social sciences.

By mid-1986, the unemployment–health link was sufficiently well established amongst non-expert opinion for new initiatives to have been undertaken whereby local authorities and health authorities in some areas set up programmes of job-creation, aiming their programmes especially at groups hardest hit by recession (see Harris and Smith 1987). Here was a new task for health education and health promotion professionals, at least, as much as this relatively small group could deal with at the time, in providing special measures to protect the health of the unemployed (Black and Laughlin 1985). And such work had, for organisational reasons, to be under the general supervision of public health doctors. There was an opportunity here for the latter to move towards some compensation of the loss of their previous 'empires', namely the local authority social work departments which had gained indepdendence under the Seebohm reforms.

There was also sufficient residual academic interest for researchers to find space in journals for occasional papers on the subject, including many participants in the earliest stages of the debate getting some 'return' on that investment (Westcott 1987; Brenner 1987a, 1987b; Forbes and Macgregor 1987; Charlton *et al.* 1987).

There were therefore several groups such as health educators and 'promoters', community development workers, and academics who could continue 'getting mileage' out of the issue as if 'the health of the unemployed' had been accepted as a legitimate problem requiring the use of their skills. At the same time as the health educators and community development workers could ignore the doubts and complexities of the academic debate, some researchers could continue to write as if the 'wearing off of selection' argument had never been proposed. For example, Forbes[1] and McGregor (who, although economists, also must be regarded as politically relatively sympathetic to the aims of those who promoted Brenner's work) wrote in 1987: 'Interpretation [of the LS results] is difficult because the researchers cannot control for the role of ill-health in generating some of the unemployment experienced by their sample', and Charlton (a statistician working for the DHSS and in terms of political background and allegiance far less sympathetic to Brenner's early sympathisers): 'LS findings ... do not rule out the possibility of a selection effect'.

Other groups now discovered new paths towards their goals and new markets for their expertise. At its first meeting in 1985 (on 16 January), an agenda item had been 'Whither UHSG?' It was felt that despite Kenneth Clarke's statement at the MIND conference:

> We [are] not 'over the top' yet as regards government attitudes, research findings and the Unemployment Health and Social Policy Report [the 'Leeds Report'] ... the steadily more conclusive findings of research needed wider dissemination ... The facts about the quality of life on the dole ... and the effects of relative poverty of the long-term unemployed (e.g. on nutrition ...) needed wider dissemination.

Even this statement, it should be noted, does not refer explicitly to any new technical argument countering the claims that the unemployed were selected for poor health, although this was the only one which had been made with any confidence. On the contrary, they rely on 'facts about ... quality of life ... and the effects of relative poverty' on health. Neither in 1985 nor to the present day has any researcher claimed to show a well-founded connection between relative poverty and quality of life and deterioration in the health of unemployed people. These ideas remain at the level of hypothesis (in, for example Wilkinson 1990). But the UHSG's April 1985 meeting was the last which was devoted mainly to the discussion of research into unemployment and health. The new direction for the Study Group was signalled by a short paragraph in the April minutes about work by Gill Westcott on 'The cost to the economy of maintaining unemployed workers'. From this point, the Study Group began to take more interest in matters such as job creation. They felt that they had been successful in wringing two ministerial admissions that unemployment 'affected health'. The first was Clarke's speech to the MIND conference. The second was in the form of a letter (dated 1 July 1985) from Secretary of State for Health and Social Security Norman Fowler to Michael Meacher (who had, at the suggestion of UHSG members, sent Fowler a copy of the Leeds Report). In the letter, Fowler stated that he 'would not question that unemployment may well have negative effects on health in many cases' and that the DHSS 'continues to monitor research evidence on the relationship between unemployment and health, to take it into account in the formulation of policy, and bring it to the attention of other government departments as appropriate'.

In a talk given to the group in February of 1986, research on how social workers, health visitors and health educators dealt with unemployed clients was given the main emphasis. This was a move towards an interest in the 'alleviation of the effects of unemployment on health' (as advocated by the government economist), and seemed to mark an upturn in interest in the Study Group. The meeting of 21 February 1986 was attended by a relatively large number of thirteen people. It seems that at this point some participants from the beginning of the debate, who had stood back from the intensely technical developments of 1982–4, now re-entered it, and aided to complete the shift from 'research dissemination' to 'service' and 'policy' issues.

From 'social' to 'technical' interest

Understanding the ways in which groups and individuals enter a debate in pursuit of a wide variety of their own objectives also clarifies an important point about the differences between the 'interest model' and the 'translation model' of the relationship between research and policy. Early 'interest' theorists gave priority to the macro-political interests of participants in scientific debates, so that at the beginning of this study a search was carried out for differences between members of the two 'sides' in social background and political sympathies.

However, Critics of the 'interest' model developed by Barnes and Bloor and applied by Mackenzie to the development of medical statistics have raised questions about the use of 'political and social interests' as candidates for the explanation of changing scientific ideas. For example, Woolgar (1981) asked what would actually count as an instance of 'interests determining knowledge'. Woolgar accuses interest-theorists of a 'general strategy ... to reveal interests as a kind of backcloth of attendant circumstances, and to imply that this revelation throws into better perspective the knowledge claim or event which is at issue'. His (and others') criticisms of studies using an 'interest model' include a disgreement with the failure to treat 'interests' as themselves resources strategically used by actors. Why should scientists' interests be regarded as some kind of latent influence on scientific work and yet 'unproblematically available to the sociologist'? And, indeed, these were some of the problems produced by the accounts given by scientists of their involvement – looking too hard for social or political factors made it harder to understand the accounts given by participants themselves of why they became active in this debate (for example 'We can do it better than they can...'). Searching for such influences in interviews produced puzzling results. Here for purposes of illustration is a description of the family background and attitudes of three leading participants in the 'unemployment and health debate', as the participants themselves spoke about them:

A: My grandfather came over here as a refugee and the family lived in the East End of London in terrible conditions – five boys all in one room ... My father was a *full-time* NHS consultant ... I am trying to improve the benefits and health of low-income people ... my concern is to be a ... social engineer.

B: I originally intended to do an economics degree so that I could go into my father's business ... seemed the most natural thing ... He always said there is no such thing as a fair profit. A fair profit is whatever profit you can get.

C: [*Political sympathies with the Liberal party, comfortable but not 'rich' family background.*] I don't believe there should be unemployment benefits at all really. I know that I would *never* sign on the dole. I'd rather do any job. If unemployment benefit wasn't there, you'd see, there'd be no more unemployment.

Here are three researchers from different social backgrounds, and with very different attitudes. It may surprise you (it certainly did me) that the first probably did more than any other individual to convince his peers that unemployment had no effect on health, the second two did as much to convince people that it did. The third produced what was generally acknowledged to be some of the most technically sound early evidence in favour of there being an effect of unemployment on health. The second wrote the most widely reported paper claiming to demonstrate a similar effect. Clearly, in this case study, it would be difficult to make a case for a strong effect of social background or political interests on the scientific stance adopted by individuals.

However, other studies have revealed the importance of other types of interest in the construction of scientific knowledge, that is 'technical interest'. By technical interest is meant the interest of occupational sub-groups in creating a continuing market for the specific techniques and forms of expertise of which they can claim 'ownership'. The contrast here is not however merely one between one type of interest and another, but also a question of how the relationship between action and interest is conceptualised. By focusing on 'technical' or 'professional' interests it became easier to see scientists (and others engaged in both academic and policy debates) 'translating' their own and each others' stock in trade in the effort to form alliances which would support each group's objectives.

Talking to researchers and others involved in the unemployment and health debate led to the conclusion that they all knew perfectly well what they were up to. However, these goals were not always stated in an open way. Strangely enough, it could probably be argued that technical interests are at least as unobtrusive as social and political ones, if not more so. This is not because professionals or scientists are not aware of them, but because the overt discussion of these matters is not considered good form. No community physician ever says outright 'We don't want to be stuck with dreary jobs like planning medical manpower and closing down small hospitals, which incur the contempt of our clinical colleagues; we'd rather have our business seen to be as important as life and death issues in clinical medicine'. No academic ever admits in so many words 'I don't want to be too critical of research team X's theory in case they referee my next grant proposal'; or, as the case may be 'I've given X's proposal the thumbs down because I don't want her team to get into that field ahead of mine.' Pursuing interests is done, often with great skill and determination, but is referred to as 'horse trading' and not often made a topic for reflection on the type of occasion represented by an interview for example. However a realisation that actors are involved in such strategies, once arrived at, makes it possible to see how ideas are offered as enrolment devices to potential allies and client groups – professional sub-groups, officials, funding bodies, and so on.

The political connection

There was a set of objectives among some participants in the unemployment and health debate which could be labelled 'political'. This was the wish of the UHSG especially its leading members, to influence Labour Party policy, and perhaps to gain individual advancement within the party.[2] In 1984 Scott-Samuel was asked by Michael Meacher to draw up a list of five people to constitute a 'front-bench advisory group' to the Shadow Cabinet on health. The group met regularly in Westminster as long as Meacher was opposition spokesperson on health. On 2 May 1986, came the first public indication that the Labour party intended to take up the health consequences of unemployment as one reason for its own economic strategy. A House of Commons press release by Meacher stated: 'Over 17,000 people have died as a result of unemployment since 1979, Michael Meacher, Labour's chief spokesman on Health and Social Services, reveals today at a North-Western TUC Health Committee'. Using Scott-Samuel's by now well-publicised extrapolation of the 1984 LS paper, Meacher claimed that 'Just over 3,000 people will die this year because of unemployment'. On 17 May, the *BMJ*'s regular 'Letter from Westminster' column was headed 'Unemployment kills, claims Labour's Michael Meacher' (Johnston 1986), validating Meacher's figure of '3,000 deaths' in 1986 as 'a statistic based on data provided by the OPCS Longitudinal Study survey of the effects of unemployment.' The Westminster columnist, Philip Johnston, comments:

> Statistical experts and medical researchers may be able to find major flaws in Mr Meacher's analysis. But to the layman – namely the ordinary voter – it is a chilling catalogue. The claims appear to be outlandish, but even if only half true they can hardly be ignored.

At the end of June, the Labour Party launched the first of a series of regional campaigns in Newcastle upon Tyne, 'The battle for jobs and welfare', stressing the health and social costs of unemployment. A member of the LS team attended a conference on unemployment and health arranged jointly by the UHSG at Manchester Town Hall in November 1986. This was the only time that any member of the group of researchers at the SSRU working on the LS data ever attended a meeting organised by the Study Group. He was greatly intrigued by the Study Group members he met, but considered the tenor of the conference 'unworldly', 'utopian' and not seriously connected with the epidemiological work on unemployment and mortality in which he was involved. But these 'utopian' topics were working very well for the Study Group, which went into 1987 with unprecedented support. Members continued to be invited to speak at meetings all over Britain, to advise on research programmes (including the ESRC's '16–19 Initiative') and talk to journalists (but now to feature writers more than 'news' reporters). This had been achieved without members gaining an understanding of 'health selection effects', or making any specific use of the more technically sophisticated arguments developed by either the medical statisticians or the economists.

The wish to change the Labour party's policies towards unemployment expressed by some early participants in the debate in the late 1970s now seemed so out of date as to be almost bizarre. Events between the General Elections of 1979 and 1987 had nearly wiped out the memory of Dennis Healey's deflationary economic policies, and of the overriding concern with inflation rather than unemployment. Those who wished to increase Labour's concern with health had a similar experience. 'Health' was second only to 'unemployment' in Labour's stated priorities in the 1987 election.

Meanwhile, 'Manifesto' community medicine and its 'social medicine' allies in academic departments found other social problems to tackle: health inequality, democracy in the NHS, equity in resource allocation, the need for more public health education at a time when the threat of AIDS seemed to loom over Britain's sexually active population (for once, health education really did seem to be a life and death matter). All these concerns could be combined, conceptually and organisationally, under the banner of the need for a New Public Health, raised initially by Peter Draper. On 26 March the *Health and Social Service Journal* published a paper jointly written by Draper and Scott-Samuel on

'Whatever happened to Public Health?' (Draper and Scott-Samuel 1986). It set out an agenda for a new 'public health militancy'. Following a serious outbreak of salmonella poisoning at Stanley Royd hospital in Wakefield, the Secretary of State for Health and Social Services, Norman Fowler, had ordered an inquiry into the role of 'public health doctors and community medicine', announced in the Commons on 20 January (Hencke 1986). Draper and Scott-Samuel used this opportunity to gain publicity for the ideas of 'Manifesto' community medicine. They called for a greater understanding of the health significance of public policy more generally, for instance, in agriculture or housing, in order to develop health enhancing rather than health damaging public policy. They claimed that: 'The conflict between free market ideology and public health is one of the reasons why a public health approach is intrinsically "political" '.[3] Copies of the *H&SSJ* article were circulated to a group of people who were then invited to begin discussions aimed at setting up a 'Public health alliance', supported also by David Player, the editorial group of *Radical Community Medicine*, and even sections of the BMA, as illustrated by two editorials in the *BMJ*, both written by Richard Smith (Smith 1986a, b).[4]

Other enterprising professional groups could also 'get mileage out of' the new social-problem processes which succeeded 'unemployment and health': the first Chair of the newly formed Public Health Alliance was the Secretary of the Health Visitors' Association, Shirley Goodwin, and the first major organisation to affiliate was the Royal College of Nursing. On the subject of new directions for community medicine, the editorial group of *Radical Community Medicine*, in the Autumn edition of 1986 (vol, 27) could see that: public health was 'beginning to be fashionable again … the Black Report [on health inequalities] is probably more relevant here than the Acheson inquiry [on the organisation of Community Medicine] looks likely to be'. Here the 'Manifesto' group more or less explicitly pose the social problem of 'health inequality' as a likely saviour of their mainstream subprofession from the threat of being re-organised out of existence. But the involvement of prominent 'Manifesto' community physicians in these new adventures left yet another gap in the scientists' network. As a result, in contrast to 1984, the UHSG had no prior knowledge of the publication of the January 1987 LS paper on unemployment and health. Scott-Samuel later remarked:

I would have told Andy Veitch that the excess mortality was 22 per cent last time [that is, for 1971–3] and 45 per cent this time, so he could say that unemployment had twice as much effect on mortality in 1981–83. By the way, that 145 was social class standardised, wasn't it ... [MB: I don't know] Oh well, but they [Moser *et al.*] do SAY that adjustment for class made little difference, so you *could* use it.

The incident gives a picture of the touch-and-go nature of enrolment processes. The professional reputation of a public health doctor does not depend on 'academic caution'. Theirs was the tradition of blowing up the cholera-infested well first, and dealing with the consequences later. The major information subsidy of the LS team's 1984 paper was due to the efforts of the UHSG, and Scott-Samuel's willingness to go into print (not without some trepidation) with a figure of 'extra deaths due to unemployment'. Being so evidently 'taken up' by a pressure group may have alarmed the scientists, or caused them to be criticised. It must be remembered that the LS researchers 'played the game according to the rules' and did not indulge in 'soap box' exercises, a strategy which enhanced the credibility of their work in the eyes of colleagues. But this decorum was only accompanied by policy impact when the researchers were linked into the network of the pressure groups. By 1987 interests had quite simply drifted in opposite directions. So there were no media-friendly re-hashes of the 1987 paper, no briefing of opposition spokespeople.

Irrelevant excellence

The reason why so much of the work on the LS looked (to me, and to other participants in the network around 'the health effects of unemployment) so 'good' and 'relevant' was that at one point it almost did provide an 'obligatory point of passage' for two major debates: on the health consequences of unemployment, and those of other social inequalities. The concept of wearing-off of selection effects was explicitly presented by Social Statistics Research Unit (SSRU) staff in various papers as an answer to problems in both these areas of inquiry. It seemed to hold the potential to close the circuit and finally bring into contact the concerns expressed, for example: at the Stirling 'consultation' of 1982; in the work of some economists since 1979 on the characteristics of the unemployed; and in the Black report, with those of campaigners on the 'single issue' of unemployment and health.

Some participants in and observers of the debate had suggested that the 'excessive' nature and 'showy' presentation of Brenner's early papers had actually damaged the cause of those who wished to carry out a 'serious' investigation of whether or not unemployment affected health. If the debate had been conducted from the beginning in a lower key, if claims had been put forward 'according to the rules' of academic scepticism, then the attention of hostile forces would not have been attracted to such intellectually fragile work. There may be some substance in this argument, which only further studies of other similar debates would clarify. However, workers in the 'strong programme' of SSK (for example, Shapin 1982) have suggested that in some cases it is the politically sensitive nature of debates which produces a more and more intricate and technical form in knowledge-claims, as a response to the strenuousness of the challenges coming from opponents. For example, Shapin has suggested that the social interests of groups of scientists should not be seen as sources of error and distortion but, on the contrary, 'the action of conflicting social interests ... may be seen as an important element in the development of bodies of knowledge valued as "interest-free"' (p. 143). He continues:

> Laboratory work becomes more and more 'technical' just in order to enrol and discipline allies, including politicians and industrialists. Its apparent independence is, consequently, precisely the result of the political work done in enrolling these allies. (Shapin 1988, p. 539)

Moser, Fox and colleagues' approach to 'the effect of unemployment on health' was necessarily a cautious one. This was partly because caution is part of the professional ideology of statisticians ('If it's surprising it's probably wrong'). It was partly because of Brenner's 'errors', and also perhaps because of the very hostility of government which many bemoaned. It is also possible to see it, as many participants did (and not only those who agreed with the basic proposition that unemployment damaged health) as a major piece of intellectual virtuosity – made all the more necessary because of the strength of opposition aroused by pressure-groups' attempts to use it in policy debate.

Statisticians' 'caution' is notorious, however, and the approach of the LS team was similar in all the subjects they tackled. At the time of the debate, the government statisticians in the OPCS (and the LS, as explained above, could not be continued without a great deal of co-operative work between SSRU and OPCS) found themselves chronically under attack due to the Rayner reviews. Produced under this type of pressure, the superiority of Moser *et al.*'s work over that of Brenner was never questioned (though by some it was apparently ignored). Yet that very technical superiority may have been produced because of the marginality of 'public health' in Britain, and the consequently more aggressive use of his ideas by those who sought a more prominent position for public health. It was the attempts by 'Manifesto' community medicine and its allies to break into policy fields by using Brenner's work which made the health of the unemployed important enough to arouse opposition. And it was this opposition which set the academic debate in train, creating the need for 'impartiality' and for technical sophistication.

Despite the indecisive outcome of the research debate, it did no harm to the individuals who took part. A short list of the career moves of some of them shows that by early 1991 Hugh Gravelle was Reader in Economics at Queen Mary College, David Jones Professor of Medical Statistics at Leicester University, Jennie Popay was Director of a new Health Research Unit in Manchester, Derek Cook had moved into Jones' previous post as senior lecturer in medical statistics at St George's hospital medical school, Richard Smith was Editor of the *British Medical Journal* and John Fox was Chief Medical Statistician for England and Wales and Deputy Director of OPCS.

Notes

1. The same John Forbes who had worked with Engelman on the unsuccessful research proposal of the early 1980s.
2. In 1985 a UHSG member asked another participant why she bothered doing such a lot of work on health for a 'fringe' political group 'when there could never be anything in it for you'.
3. It should perhaps be noted here, however, that in the winter of 1987, the Public Health Alliance which emerged from these efforts declared itself firmly 'non-political' and 'non-aligned'.
4. Smith's participation in the debate is a good example of 'entrepreneurialism' in its later stages, and the heterogeneous nature of 'network-building' in the translation of 'science' into public and policy debate. His series on 'Occupationless health' and the resulting book was not an original piece of research. It took pains to be 'fair' but did not avoid controversy. It made no contribution to the 'scientific debate' directly, and yet was as influential as any other piece of work in maintaining 'interest'. It also played a role in Smith becoming a favoured candidate for editorship of the Journal.

13

CONCLUSION: THE SOCIAL-PROBLEM PROCESS AND THE ABANDONMENT OF KNOWLEDGE

This account of the debate on unemployment and health has tried to show the ways in which entrepreneurial activities by professional and disciplinary sub-groups produced knowledge claims and attempted to establish these claims as resources to other significant groups. It has traced the formulation of the claims, and the controversy to which they gave rise, by treating the debate as a social problem process, and (for the latter part of the period) following it 'in hot blood'. The aim has not been to make judgement on the 'correctness' or 'incorrectness' of the claims, but to trace the ways in which groups in the scientific and trans-scientific environment of the researchers adopted or opposed knowledge claims, or took up a 'wait and see' position, all as part of their own occupational and micro-political strategies.

At the beginning of the process, the scientific groups involved were:

- Statisticians working on 'public health' issues, influenced or trained in the traditions of the General Register Office who regarded vital statistics as a form of social monitoring, and feared the decline of this role after the Rayner reviews.
- Economists involved in work on either health or labour market issues, with links to a government advisory role which had been less threatened than that of the statisticians by the political and administrative changes which took place during the period under study.
- Medical sociologists engaged in the more 'quantitative' types of study, but much further removed from any advisory role to departments of state.

All three of these groups sought a more prominent role in the health planning process, at a time when health planning questions were high on government agendas. Their participation in the unemployment and health debate can be understood by setting it against the kinds of claims they made about 'public health' and health service issues, within the economic, political and administrative context of the period at which the debate took place. Those disciplines whose members claimed that unemployment did affect health were the more threatened ones (medical sociology, social/medical statistics) and the professional group with whom they allied (community medicine) was similarly threatened, in its turn, not by Rayner reviews or other cuts in government funding provided for research, but by successive rounds of NHS reorganisation.

Economists, in contrast, had relatively well-established alliances with policy-makers in government departments. Some were also quietly pursuing a long-term strategy of enrolling factions within the medical profession (see Mulkay *et al.* 1987a, b). Others offered interpretations of the relationship between unemployment and physical health as 'resources' to client groups within government with the skill for which they were respected – the ability to tell whether the customer wanted 'the Black Magic or the Dairy Box'. In 1979 this involved questions about 'whether the RAWP formula should be changed to include measures of unemployment'. In 1981 it included a critique of Brenner's methods. In 1984 it was a matter of 'recommending measures of alleviation' within an accepted context of high rates of long-term unemployment. Economists made no efforts to gain media attention or to engage in pressure-group activity, and were indeed acutely embarrassed on the rare occasions on which the media did feature their work (a headline claiming 'No jobs link with ill health' was dismissed by one economist as 'What I am *supposed* to have said', see Black 1981). Much as some of the statisticians may have admired the entrepreneurialism of the economists, it was their professional socialization to emphasise accuracy. True to their 'form' as seen by civil servants, they pursued 'the truth' (which, as one remarked bitterly in late 1987, 'you are only allowed to tell this government once in your career'). Thus did different occupational cultures affect the ways in which members of the two disciplines reacted to changes in macro-economic and political climate.

The claim 'unemployment causes ill health/mortality' was brought to public and political debate by the activity of an 'intermediate body' (in Hall *et al.*'s sense) whose role was to promote informed discussion of health policy issues, and two quasi-pressure groups (one terming itself a 'study group', the other a 'forum') which provided 'subsidised' information, not only to the media, but to other entrepreneurial professionalising groups (health visitors, health educators, community workers). Yet we must remember that the membership of the USHP, the UHSG and the Social Costs of Unemployment Forum was also largely composed of members of the major sub-disciplines and sub-professions (sociology, community medicine, health education, community health development, etc). Participation in the pressure groups was one strategy by which the researchers stimulated demand for their expertise, and the professionals for their authority.

By early 1987, the 'Manifesto' community physicians and other sub-professional groups had found other issues through which to pursue their aims (some of these around a revived debate on the causes of and remedies for class inequalities in health, but of course the major new public health topic was AIDS). They more or less withdrew from the debate, leaving the social statisticians of the LS team with their painstakingly established 'structural' theory of the effects of unemployment on health which was now, for the time being at least, not a necessary resource either to pressure groups, political parties, aspiring professions, or government officials. As a result, the knowledge claim that 'the absence of "wearing-off" of mortality differences between groups supports a structural rather than an individual interpretation of health inequalities' remained a fragile object, little understood, and hardly used in public debate (see *Hansard* 23 October 1987, col. 1046 for the first, rather vague, appearance of the argument in Parliament). It is argued here that the fragility of this argument is the *consequence* of the strategic re-grouping of those involved in the unemployment and health debate. Certainly there is no evidence to support the opposite case (that the claim was dropped by the rest of the policy community because conclusive evidence against it had been accumulating). The idea was not discredited. It was merely abandoned, left in the twilight world or 'limbo phase of Downs' model of the social-problem process.

McCarthy (1986), in his study of the Child Poverty Action Group, has made illuminating use of Downs' 'stages'. He suggests three reasons why social-problem processes enter the 'fourth stage' of a 'twilight world of lesser attention and spasmodic recurrences of interest.'

1. The fact that 'some people think the issue is to big to solve'.
2. The social problem comes to be seen as confined to the 'rough' section of the working class, partly because of media treatment of the issue, and is therefore abandoned by labour organisations.
3. The 'dilettantism' of 'those who simply become bored and disenchanted by the issue and passively await the arrival of a new ... issue'. Here 'those' include Ministers, civil servants, academics and journalists, as well as 'middle class do-gooders' who 'flippantly desert' issues, leaving them 'largely unresolved' (pp. 100– 104).

By mid-1987, all three of these things seemed to have happened to the unemployment and health debate. Civil servants had long regarded the 'problem' as 'too big', either inherently ('what could the DHSS do about it?'), or because it crossed departmental boundaries, or because of government policy ('You know and I know this government is not going to make a U-turn'). Seaton (1986, p. 19) found that as unemployment increased during the 1980s, its news value tended to fall. Her study of coverage in *The Times* showed an 'inverse relationship between the percentage of the population out of work and the front page attention given to the subject.' One journalist, commenting on the failure of the Labour Party to take up Steve Platt's research in 1983, remarked that unemployment and suicidal behaviour was 'too big' for a political party as well. Opposition politicians, Bryan Christie felt, look for issues over which they can quickly demonstrate the superiority of their own policies. The spirit in which the likelihood of the existence of 'the unemployment effect' was admitted by a policy adviser in late 1984 had been almost one of breathlessness at the enormity of what it entailed. This was also reflected in a *Lancet* leading article of November 1984, which, perhaps unintentionally, highlighted the contrast between the (relatively) minute sums that could be spent on even the most expensive research, and what would be necessary to tackle the underlying problem of mass unemployment. Those who dealt with this larger problem in terms of practical economics had never joined in the debate on 'health'.

The second cause to which McCarthy attributes the languishing of a social problem process, that is, of the better-off and poorer sections of the working class being turned against each other, amounts to what I have termed 'moral fragmentation'. Those who suffer serious misfortune come to be seen as possessing (or lacking) quasi-moral characteristics of one kind or another. In McCarthy's case study, the misfortune is poverty rather than unemployment, but the same analysis can be applied. For McCarthy, the media play a decisive role in individualising social problems. Seaton (1986, p. 28) disagrees, and holds that the media 'have not been an overriding independent influence on attitudes towards unemployment' but rather acted as a 'catalyst' of new attitudes which emerged, as she sees it, mysteriously. This mystery may however be somewhat clarified by looking at how the British labour market operates.

Although Seaton and McCarthy attribute changes in attitudes to unemployment to 'public opinion', there may be a more concrete reason for the reduction of interest in unemployment. As the economists who took part in the debate (Stern 1979 for example) and some other social scientists who kept their distance (Sinfield 1981, Hakim 1982) were aware, the British labour market is 'segmentedl'. Low pay and the risk of unemployment are concentrated in certain sectors of industry and regions. By 1983– 4, the pattern of unemployment was one of increasing inequality of distribution : that is, the risk of unemployment was, if anything, more concentrated within social classes IV and V than it had been in the mid-1970s (Sinfield 1987), and not even throughout these social classes, but in certain segments within them. There were grounds for thinking that the tendency described by Stern for the 1970s had become even stronger as unemployment rose and then stabilised at new heights. Long-term unemployment rose far more than short-term, that is, it was not that a lot more people were experiencing short periods of joblessness, but a slightly larger number than prevously were experiencing much longer spells. As more of the total amount of unemployment was experienced by the same people, either as long-term spells without work or as a life 'in and out of work', those in steady jobs had every reason to feel less personally preoccupied by what unemployment might do to them if it struck.

In the present case study other factors also seem to have been at work in reducing 'the health of the unemployed' to the level of an individual problem. The media did not play a major part in this. Although newspapers occasionally picked up statements made by those who opposed the idea that unemployment affected health ('Dole is like a holiday, says economist'), 'Death on the dole' headlines were the vast majority. We need to look elsewhere for the source of individualisation, and this study has argued that it was the entrepreneurial activities of some economists, their established alliances and the new enrolments which they sought, which produced an account of the poor health of the unemployed as a product of individual characteristics. Changes in public awareness and perception of the phenomenon of unemployment in Britain may well have played a role in the easy acceptance of these experts' views, however. As labour market trends became clearer, it was less and less likely that labour organisations would ever be 'enrolled' in a debate on the health of the unemployed (although they began to take up the question of the pay and conditions of workers in the 'secondary labour market'). At the same time, sociologists were showing that there was a growth in the proportion of the labour force employed in low-paid, part-time, and/or intermittent forms of work (Fevre 1986, Walker, Noble and Westergaard 1985, Harris, Lee and Morris 1985, Martin 1987). Unions organising unskilled and service sector workers, as well as some industrial and urban sociologists, could have been 'enrolled' by those researchers who believed there were impor-tant health consequences to recession, and who wrote of 'residualisation' as did Fox (1986 unpublished), Moser *et al.* (1987a), and Platt (1986b). But the difficulties involved in sus-taining any form of 'enrolment' between reforming groups and the 'unskilled' working class, the unemployed, or other consum-ers of social welfare services has been commented upon, for ex-ample, by Hall *et al.* (1978, p. 91), and Ditch (1986).

This unfulfilled possibility is the reason why McCarthy's third point, on 'dilettantism' needs to be considered rather more carefully as it applies to the present case study. Firstly, the considerations of 'time', priorities, and funding which have been discussed in Part II indicate that we can perhaps go beyond a concept of 'dilettantism' in explaining why expert groups abandon social problems. Aca-demics, for example, must enrol resource holders if they wish to acquire the means to do research of any kind. Secondly, although necessary discretion exercised by both academics funded by gov-ernment departments and by civil servants created considerable problems in interpreting some of what was said in interviews and other 'formal' occasions, questions about the degree of 'pressure' applied to unruly experts have to be addressed. Only a fine line divides the ability to 'see whether the customer wants the Milk

Tray or the Dairy Box' from 'government suppression of research', and some field material did indicate that certain researchers felt under considerable pressure to abandon work on the effects of social inequality and unemployment on health. The spirit of routinely 'moving on to the next thing' certainly influenced some who decided to drop unemployment and health as a topic.[1] Others, however, by 1987, did seem discouraged even to the extent of feeling a sense of 'depression' and futility, which, they feared, had affected their intellectual productivity.

There were some, certainly, who felt that the community physicians who became involved in the debate had been engaged on an imperialistic exercise, and who might therefore regard their loss of interest as a form of opportunism (such as that attributed to medical sociologists by Strong, 1979) or 'dilettantism'. This would, however, be rather a simplified picture of the way in which entrepreneurial sub-professions dealt with unemployment and health. 'Manifesto' community physicians such as Peter Draper had always made it clear that the topic was not central to them but only one issue which could be used as a vehicle to promote wider objectives. Like academics, civil servants (including professional advisers) and journalists, as has been discussed, have a 'cycle of credibility' which involves 'having a bright idea and fighting for it', and then 're-investing' the career capital thus obtained. If there is dillettantism or opportunism, it must be regarded as institutional in nature.

The decline of interest amongst sub-professional factions, for example within medicine, social work, community health development, and health education did, however, have an important effect on the academic debate. This interest had reached its peak in 1981–2, and been reflected in the rush of conferences on unemployment and health which had encouraged groups such as the UHSG and SCUF, and produced a high demand for their expertise. Since that time, however, other events had intervened to increase the confidence with which these professionalising groups could enter new territories. During 1981–2, to judge from the content of their Annual Conferences, health visitors, and even librarians, for example, were adopting the welfare of the unemployed as a legitimate area for the exercise of their skills. But by 1986 it was no longer necessary for these groups to enter into debates over the *knowledge*-claim that unemployment damaged health. The knowledge claim was either sufficiently accepted by decision-makers within the professions and their organisational contexts, or far less important as they found new reasons to claim a portion in the wider social problem of unemployment. As the sub-professional groups lost interest in the subject, journalists were no longer receiving 'information subsidy' on it. And *it was the disappearance of this phenomenon – sub-professional activism combined with information subsidy which lowered the political temperature of the academic debate.* No longer a 'political hot potato', unemployment and health no longer attracted resources on the 'customer–contractor' or 'concordat' (see Chapter 11) principles by which government Departments could persuade scientifically respectable groups to devote resources to 'fuzzy' topics.

Implications for theory and method

The objective of this study was to take some steps in developing the way in which the relationship between research and policy debates are understood. To do this, concepts have been adopted from both social policy and the sociology of science and technology. In attempting to understand the progress of a policy-related academic controversy, and thereby to better understand the shifting status of the factual claims which it may produce, the concepts and methods of the 'Strong Programme' in the sociology of scientific knowledge have proved valuable. By giving equal weight to all knowledge claims, devoting equal attention to those regarded as 'true' and 'false' and seeking the social and organisational patterns which give rise to both 'rational' and 'irrational' beliefs this method allows a common perspective to be applied to studying the actions of researchers and policy actors ('authorities and partisans' in the words of Hall *et al.*). An established 'fact' in a policy-related inquiry is just one possible outcome of a social problem process. 'Facts' occur when statements become 'obligatory points of passage' that bind together a variety of those groups which have entered the process seeking their own different objectives. Recent studies of policy communities (for example, McMahon *et al.* 1983) and their interaction with researchers offer a very similar analysis to those of the sociologists of science whose work has been used as a guide in this study. For example, speaking of social research in government, Walker (1987) feels that:

> it would be wrong to underestimate the individual motives and sub-departmental interests that underpin some government research. In the same way that researchers may initiate

research to further their own individual and collective interest, so do policy-makers ... As a result, policies tend to
evolve ... in part at least – through a process of conflict and
changing alliances between policy divisions in which research
is one of the many 'weapons' that are deployed.

Describing the wider context of such Whitehall dealings, Moon
and Richardson point out that: 'Virtually all political issues carry
with them a constellation of groups, jockeying to influence policy-
makers ... and trying to influence the definition of the issue to
their own advantage'. Groups are engaged in pursuing a wide
variety of objectives, and knowledge-claims are a currency
(amongst others) in this process. A knowledge claim which
proves useful to the all relevant groups becomes an 'obligatory
point of passage' and is accepted as 'fact'. Scientific debates will
persist when unadjudicated claims create bottle-necks which
hinder either the accomplishment of professional or political objectives (which, as we have seen, are often closely inter-related).
But debates do not only end in closure by the establishment of
'facts'. They can also end when the participants *simply disengage*,
when other means of reaching groups' objectives become available. Under these circumstances potential points of passage become mere diversions or dead ends, and knowledge claims no
longer attract even enough attention to sustain controversy.

There are other examples of (at least temporarily] abandoned
knowledge claims, such as the outcomes of debate on race or class
and intelligence (Harwood 1979, 1982), and of the investigation of
environmental hazards such as lead or radiation. What is the
current epistemological status of the factual claims made in the
course of these debates? In terms of the 'translation' approach to
the sociology of science, the question is not whether some are true
and others false, but rather what were the organisational and
political circumstances which gave rise to these claims and what
changes in these circumstances led to the ending of controversy?
This may result from the judicial decision at the end of an inquiry,
for example, or a reorganisation of the school system brought
about following a change of government. Such questions are per-
tinent (according to the 'rule of symmetry') whether or not one
aspect of this closure of debate was an acceptance of the truth of
specific knowledge-claims.

In conclusion, to return to the set of questions of theory and
method posed at the beginning of this account, can approaches

derived from the sociology of scientific knowledge and a 'social problems' perspective help to organise the material produced in a case study such as the present one in such a way as to aid in understanding its progress? How well did concepts taken from these two perspectives 'fit' the unfolding events in the debate? Can we analyse the relationship between social research and social policy in a similar way to that used to understand the relationship between science and technology?

This study aimed to follow a policy-related academic debate 'in hot blood', to see whether what some onlookers and participants (including myself) saw at the time (late 1982) as academically superior research would have a greater impact on policy discussion and decision-making than the 'discredited' work of M. H. Brenner. The present account has been structured by the attempt to apply a social-problems perspective elaborated according to the 'translation' model of the construction of scientific knowledge. Material has been selected by a series of decisions taken on the basis of the theoretical approaches adopted. These approaches, however, were not adopted at the beginning of the study and carried throughout. Early theoretical approaches were tentatively applied and, in many cases, had to be rejected, sometimes after a lengthy process involving the collection of much material, which ended up as one or two sentences. For example, I felt that the prediction that media interest in the health aspects of unemployment would be aroused by spates of factory closure stories, marches of the unemployed, or other similar 'macro-social' events could be regarded as discredited only after some two years of collecting newspaper cuttings, pressure-group minutes, and notes from Hansard. This finding increased my confidence in the idea that the social-problem process in this case was created by entrepreneurial activities amongst sub-professional and sub-disciplinary groups . But to see it as a 'positive' finding *in support* of my analysis is to ignore my earlier 'hunches' about the role played by 'the media reacting to social movements and macro-economic change' as a force in the social-problem process. The reluctance of the media to follow up plant closures with 'health' stories appeared, at first, as something as puzzling as the insistence of a high proportion of my scientists that they were totally uninterested in the health effects of unemployment full stop, and even more so in whatever 'political' meaning the debate might be seen as having.

Nor was this study begun with the aim of 'integrating' the social-problems and translation perspectives. At first, the two approaches appeared to apply to quite separate aspects of the debate. Interview and field material relevant to the scientific controversy was addressed with the aid of concepts drawn from the 'translation' model as described in Chapters 1 and 8. The social-problem 'stages' model was used to make sense of the policy debate and the material derived from interviews with officials, activists, and media-workers. As both the history of the debate and the progress of the interviewing continued, however, there were two developments.

Firstly, it began to be clear that there were more similarities than I had expected between the ways in which members of the different groups involved in the debate spoke about their own actions. Secondly, a new literature began to emerge in the sociology of scientific knowledge, which seemed to point to a convergence between ways of understanding 'pure' scientists, and ways of understanding 'technologists' administrators, and even 'politicians'. Sociologists of scientific knowledge (this is the point of not calling the perspective 'sociology of science') had long insisted that the cognitive closure of scientific debates could only be accounted for in terms of the social relationships within which science is located. The data in the present study stubbornly refused to display social or political interests as characteristics decisively differentiating the antagonists in the debate. This led to increasing concentration on the professional rather than the political allegiance of participants, and on the micro-politics of what seemed to be the relevant 'technology' namely, 'social engineering', the technologies of welfare .

The results of using these two approaches in the study of a policy-related academic debate can be summarised:

1. *The social problem perspective* not only provided a useful guide to the overall progress of the debate (the 'stages'), but also clarified aspects of the scientific process *within* the debate. In fact, the 'translation' approach itself can usefully be regarded as a type of social-problem perspective.

A 'stages model' derived from the social-problems perspective, and Spector and Kitsuse's method of 'following the problem wherever it goes' both guides the researcher through the debate and helps to order the material which results. However, as Manning has pointed out, the 'stages model' requires to be adapted and elaborated by a more detailed understanding of the different groups which become involved in social problem processes. In the present study this has involved drawing concepts from other work, such as Gandy's on the media, Richardson and Jordan, Heclo and Wildavsky, and Lindblom on the operation of 'issue communities', and sociologists of scientific knowledge on science as a socially-organised activity.

Useful concepts derived from work using this approach included *'moral* and *technical fragmentation'*, as described by Manning. A similar process in the unemployment and health debate as that described by Manning's account of the Mental Health Act of 1982 (Manning 1985, pp. 20– 2) did seem to take place. However, events seemed to call for a rather more complex application of the concepts. 'Technical fragmentation' was seen to be a response to strong contestation of a political and/or academic type (or, more accurately, to the type of powerful academic counterargument which could be produced given a decision by policymakers to 'interest' academics in investing time and effort in such an argument). Rather differently to what is proposed by Habermas (1972, and see also discussion of this by Scott 1988) and some of his followers, the present study did not find that technical fragmentation operated as a form of social control exerted by or through scientists. On the contrary, the more technically fragmented an argument became, the more likely it was that all sides of a policy debate would eventually lose interest in it.

'Moral fragmentation' could take place at higher or lower levels of technical sophistication and was independent of this. Moral fragmentation comes closer to the concepts used both by Habermas and by Manning, that is, the 'reduction' of a collective problem to one concerned with the characteristics of individuals.

2. In exploring the *role of the media* in the debate, the concept of *'information subsidy'* was found extremely useful. The role of the media was not at all what had been expected at the outset of the study . Rather than any consistent tendency of journalists independently to distort or sensationalise research results and other forms of expert pronouncement, it appeared that experts' attempts to 'interest' client groups and to claim a role in the social problem process played a major role, through the mechanism of information subsidy, in producing media stories which attracted public attention

3. Ideas about where 'pressure groups' were to be found had

to be revised. Here the work of Lindblom and Walker (1987) was illuminating. As a social-problems perspective would lead us to expect, entrepreneurial 'ginger groups' were not only present within professions, disciplines and government departments, but provided in this case at least, an important part of the impetus which resulted in the reconstruction of what was 'relevant' 'valid' and so on. The first hint of this was the difficulty I had when coding my interviews, as described in Chapter 9. The initial distinction between 'authorities' and 'partisans' was far too simple to be maintained throughout the case study. For one thing, the most energetic members of pressure groups were also enterprising professionals or academics, and not (as may be the case in other social-problem processes) members of wider social movements.

4. *Understanding scientists.* There were two rather different approaches to the sociology of science used in this study. The first I have called an 'interest model' and the second a 'translation model'. Both contributed important concepts and methodological procedures.

The *'translation' approach* added a vital resource to the process of attempting to understanding the actions of scientists. Rather more surprisingly, concepts drawn from this new perspective in the sociology of scientific knowledge were illuminating when considering the actions of officials and professionals, both in the 'more' and 'less academic' phases of the debate. This might have been expected, given that the chosen debate was one with a high 'scientific' content.

As discussed above, the study began with an expectation that 'social and/or political interests' of scientists would be found to influence their approach to the question of whether unemployment causes ill-health. This expectation was not borne out fully as interviewing and field work progressed. However, the 'interest model' forced the study to look beyond the 'interests' only of non-scientists; for example, it does not encourage the researcher to expect that 'only politicans or pressure groups have interests' and that science proceeds in a cultural vacuum. 'Interests' play an important role in the framing, contestation, and acceptance of knowledge claims as 'fact'. However, in the present study, neither social background nor political allegiance seemed to account fully for participants' actions. In addition, it was necessary to understand the 'interest-work' carried out by individuals as members of entrepreneurial sub-professional or sub-disciplinary groups, and the relationships of these groups to each other and to other, often similarly 'entrepreneurial' client-groups.

From the work of Latour and Woolgar and of Knorr-Cetina came the valuable notion of 'cycles of credibility' in the scientific career. This is another concept which proved usable beyond its original territory. In the process of tracing the 'stages' of social problem claims-making, it has emerged that scientists, journalists, professionals and officials can all be regarded as following the 'cycles of credibility' appropriate to their occupational cultures. In order to understand *who* becomes involved in policy-related academic debates, these aspects of occupational culture need to be addressed. In order to understand what those who become involved do, it is necessary to trace out the objectives of the groups involved, and the ways in which individuals and groups pursue these objectives by 'inter-esting' and forming alliances with each other.

An important contribution of the translation model was its clearly-laid-out *concepts* and *rules of method*. These have guided the analysis of the activities of individual members of the debate's 'core group' and of the professional and disciplinary factions to which they belonged. The two principles of *'beginning with controversy'* and *'following the course of action wherever it leads'* are common to both Latour and Callon's translation perspective and Spector and Kitsuse's method for the investigation of social problem processes. Adherence to these rules of method was more or less inevitable given the starting point of the present study. The 'principle of *symmetry*' helped to avoid attempts to 'fix' the state of knowledge in the debate at any given point in time as having established what was 'really the case', which would have been a fruitless exercise and might have cut off the investigation arbitrarily. The principle of *'explanation by association and situation'* has helped to concentrate the analysis on the shifting balance of alliances between scientists, professionals and officials which gave the debate its shape. We have seen in this account the varying degrees to which sub-disciplines concentrated on 'translating' their theories, methods and findings into forms which would attract allies from their trans-scientific fields, and the outcome of these efforts in terms of research coming to be seen as more or less 'policy-relevant' 'fundable' and 'yielding firm results'.

However, as outlined above, the translation approach does benefit from insights drawn from the social-problems perspective, and needs to be further developed by other case studies involving more detailed consideration of the dynamics at work in the 'trans-scientific field' of government departments, funding bodies, professions and wider social movements.

One aspect of the enrolment process made more visible in the present case-study than it may have been in some others (for example, Callon 1986, Coutouzis and Latour 1985) is the effect of science policies formulated at governmental level and acting via decisions made in the 'independent' research councils. The effect of the Rothschild reforms in encouraging research councils to look favourably upon 'policy-relevant' work was to raise the priority of 'unemployment and health' in the eyes of MRC-funded research teams . As well as making it 'controversial', the political salience of the debate also made it 'policy-relevant'. This had consequences for scientists' opportunities to advance their own individual 'cycles of credibility' and those of the research groups they belonged to.

As Collins (1985) has warned, attracting more attention is a double-edged weapon to a research team. New allies (as Latour 1987 also points out) can be unreliable, and new opponents may also be attracted into the field. However, as Shapin (1982) has argued, conflict also intensifies scientists' efforts to construct their claims as 'objective' and 'value-free'. The knowledge-claim 'the effect of unemployment on mortality cannot be due to selection' was based on an intricate argument. This argument expressed a tentative 'lash-up' of several professional and disciplinary sub-groups: public-health oriented medical statisticians and community physicians, occupational medicine, vital statisticians concerned with 'social indicators' (another group which might have been expected to be included was the 'poverty lobby', but by late 1987 this enrolment had not yet been seriously attempted from either side: researchers' or activists'). Whether this statement would become a 'fact' depended (and continued to depend at the end of the study period) on the strength of the associations and alliances around the researchers. Between September 1986 and late 1987 these alliances appeared to become 'untied', and the 'wearing off of selection' began to fade towards uncertainty. But it does not by any means follow that the statement will not, at some future time, regain a degree of 'solidity', if it once again provides a potential 'point of passage' through which a sufficient number of interest-groups must pass in pursuit of their aims, and if these aims are met with 'success' in policy terms. In the unlikely event, for example, of a marked equalisation of living and working conditions in British society being followed by a reduction in class inequalities in mortality, the ideas developed at the Social Statistics Research Unit might well come to be regarded as unquestioningly as those of John Snow on cholera (Jones and Cameron 1983) or Pasteur on anthrax (Latour 1984b). It is, however, as pointed out by the economist in Chapter 6, most unlikely that such policy change would come about *because* the arguments of any particular group of researchers were 'accepted'.

Reformulating the relationship between research and policy

This argument returns us to the question of the relationship between the 'quality' of research (as judged by the 'scientific community') and its impact on policy debate. Bulmer (1986) points out that in Cohen and Garet's (1975) study of the effect of applied social research on educational policy-making: 'There was no clear connection between relevance, methodological sophistication and authoritativeness [partly because] methodologically superior knowledge was more complex, arcane and hard to interpret'. In the course of the debate described by Cohen and Garet, as in the present case study: 'the knowledge produced improved by any scientific standard, but was not more authoritative by any political standard, and often more mystifying by any public standard' (Bulmer 1986, p. 26–7).

Latour makes an observation on this point which is highly relevant to anyone concerned with the public image of science and the dissemination of scientific ideas:

> popularisation follows the same route as controversy but in the opposite direction; it was because of the intensity of the debates that we were … led from non-technical sentences [and] large numbers of ill-equipped verbal contestants to small numbers of well-equipped contestants … *It is hard to popularise science because it is designed to force out most people in the first place.* (1987, p. 52)

In the debate described here, and perhaps in others, the more numerous but poorly equipped verbal contestants from the pressure groups and political movements seem to have played such an important role that without them the efforts of the scientists threatened to be in vain. The constant struggle between being technical enough to fend off scientific competitors and not too technical to persuade policy-makers and opinion leaders of the value of what researchers do arises from the very heart of the social construction of knowledge.

However, it cannot be concluded from this study of the unemployment and health debate that there is necessarily a trade-off between 'quality equals complexity' on the one hand and 'clarity equals over-simplification' on the other. Brenner's work was regarded as the most 'arcane' by participants, though not as the 'best'. Nor can the failure of the LS team's work to become widely accepted be attributed to its complexity alone. While there was no shortage of higly technical work on both sides of this debate, that by economists was seen to be relatively easily translatable into one stance in policy terms, whereas that by statisticians was not readily accessible to those who took opposing views. The entrepreneurial genius of the economists was to translate their sophisticated mathematical models into policy prescriptions than were both acceptable *and understandable* to the 'policy gatekeepers' (in Tizard's terms). The failing of the statisticians, cumulating in a paper (never published) by Fox and Goldblatt which expressed the wearing-off of selection in terms of a Markov chain, was that *their* technical defence of their position never became translatable into terms accessible to potential allies. And one reason for this was that the commitment to scepticism and neutrality was so deeply a part of their professional ideology. The very rules they played by, which made statistics rather than economics the centre of a 'government fiddles figures' discourse, made them equally wary of any involvement with pressure groups or political parties.

The perspectives used in this study should perhaps lead to a re-formulation of questions such as "What is the influence of research on policy?' or "Is the lack of influence of social research on policy due to the poor quality of the research?" It might be more fruitful to inquire into the ways in which 'social-problem processes' produce opportunities for claims to expertise to be made, and thereby shape both 'debated' and 'accepted' knowledge itself. Such a reformulation has been suggested by Rein, who sees the relationship as an 'interplay' (Rein 1980). Such a reformulation would bring us closer to the ways in which participants in policy-related academic debates themselves see the relationship – as constructed within an iterative process in which individuals and groups make claims about the 'truth' and 'policy-relevance' of some aspect of their work. They do this as a form of strategic advance into a new field or market-place which has opened up as a result of conflict and change in the policy making arena. Claims-making is therefore adapted to the different perceived characteristics of the field, such as the nature and strength of the opposition, and the 'interests' of potential allies. The success of know-ledge claims, and their promotion to the status of fact, depends not only on the technical skills of participants, but also on their strategic skills. Knowledge claims weave their way in and out of policy debates, often by means of such 'vectors' as research-ers' tactical use of information subsidy to the media, and partici-pation in pressure groups. Other tactics (less visible to an outside investigator and therefore not discussed at length here) include informal contact with decision-makers, as evidenced by officials' nervousness about 'stirring-up' members of the academic com-munity who are seen as able to mobilise either the media or 'powerful acquaintances'.[2] Future case studies may examine the fate of other knowledge-claims in relation to their articulation with policy objectives in this more 'symmetrical' fashion.

Outcomes of the interactions between the parties to a debate could also be seen in terms of quite transparently 'political' objec-tives: pressure groups 'wanted something to beat the government over the head with', or 'Ministers didn't want to know'. However, both the present case study, and much existing literature on Brit-ish policy-making shows that (unlike many of the participants in the debate), the sociological analyst should not simply assume that a social-democratic government is sympathetic to research and a conservative one less so. McCarthy (1986) argues that the 'right-wing research institutes' had a strong influence on Con-servative economic and social policy, by virtue of persistent and painstaking lobbying for certain ideas over a long period of time.

As we have seen, knowledge claims are produced and elabor-ated by individuals and groups with their *own* aims and objec-tives, not reactive in any simple sense to 'political pressures'. Understanding political allegiances seems to be less helpful than understanding the ways in which expert groups enter policy de-bates with a history of participation in previous social-problem processes, which has established their methods and the data available to them as 'resources'. However else are we to make sense of a paper on the health of the unemployed being produced by a study of water hardness (the British Regional Heart Study)? Or by the question appearing in a monograph intended to deal with 'the numerator-denominator question' in vital statistics (the OPCS Longitudinal Study)?

The answers to these questions lie in the histories of the studies. The possibilities open to the Regional Heart Study team were mainly determined by a series of extraordinary happenstances. The distribution of unemployment in Britain rather closely mirrors the distribution of water quality: soft water areas tend to have high unemployment.[3] In addition, there was the presence of three peripheral members of the department with interests in 'social issues'. The statisticians of the OPCS were steeped in the reforming public health traditions inherited from nineteenth-century figures such as Chadwick, Farr and Simon (Eyler 1979, Wohl 1883). They were also constrained by the very nature of their data. Censuses in Britain do not contain questions on either morbidity or health related behaviour such as smoking, drinking and exercise. Even if they had wished to, therefore, the LS researchers could not have addressed questions about whether high mortality or morbidity in unemployed men was due to pre-existing psychological ill health or to behaviour.

Nor was there anything inevitable about the prominent role played on the 'other side' of the debate by the economists. There are plenty of able sociologists and psychologists working in government departments who carry out 'defensive briefing' on politically sensitive research, yet none of these wrote major criticisms of the work of Brenner or any of his British 'sympathisers'. Conversely there were economists such as Howard Cox, Chris Pond (who had worked at the Civil Service College) and others who were at least partly sympathetic to Brenner's ideas. Those who became 'interested' in opposing Brenner's ideas seem to have been involved in wider debates on 'the determinants of health' and the relative importance in this of social conditions versus individual behaviour and genetic inheritance ('personal characteristics'). Whether or not the enrolment between certain economists and policy-makers would hold remained to be seen by the end of this case study.

The work of the LS team presented a potential challenge to the economists' alliances, because they offered a method of testing the importance of personal characteristics in certain kinds of studies. But knowledge claims about the effects of unemployment and class inequality on health did not *determine* the outcome of these attempts. On the contrary, the truth-status of the various 'findings'

and 'models' was a *result* of the varying success of the groups that
made them in enrolling allies and maintaining their alliances. An
impression was growing by the end of field work that the threat
to the size of the market for the economists' skills posed by successive waves of government re-organisations was making the
enrolment between economists and policy-makers (in this and in
other issue communities) increasingly tenuous. Booth (1982), for
example, has observed that:

> Social planning is in the doldrums ... After all, who needs to
> bother with planning if the market, released from the distor-
> tions and burdens of state intervention, official regulation
> and bureaucratic red tape, will by itself maximize national
> wellbeing?

And Michael Heseltine, during his first spell as Secretary of State
for the environment, was reputed (by disconsolate government
statisticians) to have said, 'Research on housing? We don't need
research, we take decisions on housing and we implement them,
that's all there is to it'. Such trends in government thinking were
more likely to encourage an alliance between the expert groups
themselves (for an example, see Bartley 1990).

One criterion by which to judge the usefulness of the present
study would be whether it could equip future sociologists better
to address questions about other teams of experts, such as the
'right-wing' Institutes (Adam Smith, Economic Affairs) and the
'non-aligned' ones (Brookings, PSI), and their relationships to
political parties and to Whitehall, Westminster, or Capitol Hill. A
most interesting example is recently provided by Anna Pollert's
analysis of the concept of the 'flexible firm' as a product of the
mediating role between government and industry played by an
'intermediate body', the Institute of Manpower Studies (Pollert
1987). The origins of the unemployment and health debate can be
seen, on one level, as residing in the much grander conflict in
which counter-Keynesian economic thinkers sought to mobilise
behind their technical claims (translated into the form of
'scrounger debates' for example), a growing social movement,
that is, the growing discontent with the failures of mixed
economy 'welfarism'.[4] The outcome of the present study would
suggest that future research on the question of the relationship
between research and policy might consider more carefully the
positions of professional and disciplinary sub-groups as 'entrepreneurial' claimants to areas of expertise, and of both political

parties and government officials as 'brokers' of social-problem areas.

Notes

1. Though it should be asked why the history of science contains so many instances of problems being abandoned for no immediately obvious reason (see for example Collins and Pinch 1979, p. 239) this question cannot be addressed here and 'moving on' is taken to be a routine practice.

2. For example, one leading researcher was described as having unnerved officials by attending meetings accompained by a 'minder' with powerful friends amongst Ministers.

3. It was pointed out by a member of the Water Research Centre staff that this was not so surprising. Some of the oldest industrial towns were established in soft water areas because of the needs of the textile industry. These were amongst the older heavy industries most affected by both the 1930s and 1980s recessions.

4. This would account for the attractiveness to some on *both* sides of the debate of the ideas on M. H. Brenner, which bore the mark of his early training as an economist in the Keynesian tradition.

BIBLIOGRAPHY

Acheson, E. D. (1967) *Medical Record Linkage* (Oxford: Oxford University Press).

Acheson, E. D. (1968) 'Social and medical statistics – some remarks on contemporary British medical statistics', *Journal of the Royal Statistical Society*, series A, 131: 10–28.

Acton, T. (1984) 'From public health to national health: the escape of environmental health officers from medical supervision and the fragmentation of nineteenth century concepts of health', *Radical Community Medicine*, 19: 12–23.

Akehurst, R. L. (1981) 'Health economists and the NHS: a comment' *Community Medicine*, 3: 149–53.

Allen, R. (1970) 'On official statistics and official statisticians', *Journal of the Royal Statistical Society*, series A, 133: 509–22.

Altheide, D. and J. Johnson (1980) *Bureaucratic Propaganda* (Boston: Allyn and Bacon).

Armstrong, R. (1973) 'Management training for statisticians and opportunities to enter top management', *Journal of the Royal Statistical Society*, Series A, 136: 95.

Aronson, N. (1982a) 'Nutrition as a social problem: a case study of entrepreneurial strategy in science', *Social Problems*, 29: 474–87.

Aronson, N. (1982b) 'Science as a claims-making activity: implications for social problems research' (MS, Northwestern University, USA).

Ashmore, M., Mulkay, M., and T. Pinch (1989) *Health and Efficiency* (Milton Keynes: Open University Press).

Ashworth, J. T. M. (1984) 'Science policy in the UK: a view from the centre', in M. Gibbons, P. Gummett, and B. M. Udgaonkar (eds) *Science and Technology Policy in the 1980s and Beyond* (London: Longman, 1984)

Banks, G. T. (1979) 'Programme budgeting in the NHS', in T. A. Booth (ed.) *Planning for Welfare* (Oxford: Basil Blackwell/Martin Robertson).

Banting, K. (1979) *Poverty, Politics and Policy* (Massachusetts: MIT Press).

Barnes, B. (1977) *Interests and the Growth of Knowledge* (London: Routledge and Kegan Paul).

Barnes, B. (1982) 'The Science-technology relationship: a model and query', *Social Studies of Science*, 12: 166–72.

Bartley, M. (1985) '"Coronary" health disease and the public health', *Sociology of Health and Illness*. 7: 289–313

M. Bartley (1987) 'Research on unemployment and health in Great Britain', in D. Schwefel, P. G. Svensson, and H. K. Zollner (eds) *Unemployment, Health and Social Vulnerability in Europe* (Munich: Springer-Verlag).

Bartley M. (1988) 'Unemployment and health – selection or causation: A false antithesis?', *Sociology of Health and Illness*, 10: 42–67.

Bartley, M. (1990) 'The story of r₂', in I. Varcoe, M. Macneil, and S. Yearley (eds) *Deciphering Science and Technology* (London: Macmillan).

Bartley, M. (1991) 'Health and labour force participation: stress, selection and the reproduction costs of labour power', *Journal of Social Policy*, 20: 327–64.

Beale, N. (1986) 'From brainwave to breakfast television', *British Medical Journal*, 292: 869–70.

Beale, N. and S. Nethercott (1985) 'Job loss and family morbidity: a study of factory closure', *Journal of the Royal College of General Practitioners*, 280: 510–14.

Beale, N. and S. Nethercott (1986a) 'Job-loss and health – the influence of age and previous morbidity', *Journal of the Royal College of General Practitioners*, 36: 261–4.

Beale, N. and S. Nethercott (1986b) 'Job-loss and morbidity in a group of employees nearing retirement age', *Journal of the Royal College of General Practitioners*, 36: 265–6.

Beale, N. and S. Nethercott (1986c) 'Job-loss and morbidity in married men with and without young children', *Journal of the Royal College of General Practitioners*, 36: 557–9.

Beale, N. and S. Nethercott (1986d) 'Job-loss and morbidity: the influence of job-tenure and previous work history', *Journal of the Royal College of General Practitioners*, 36: 560–63.

Beale, N. and S. Nethercott (1986e) 'From brainwave to breakfast television', *BMJ*, 292: 869–70.

Beale, N. and S. Nethercott (1987) 'The health of industrial employees four years after compulsory redundancy', *Journal of the Royal College of General Practitioners*, 37: 390–94.

Benjamin, W. (1984) 'Statistics by or for government?', *The Professional Statistician*, 3: 11.

Bijker, W. E, Hughes, T. P., and T. J. Pinch (eds) (1987) *The Social Construction of Technological Systems* (Cambridge, Mass.: MIT Press).

Black, D. K. (1986) 'The MRC and Health Services Research', paper to Welcome Unit for the History of Medicine conference: The MRC and the Development of a National Biomedical Research Policy, 8 March, 1986.

Black, D. and S. Laughlin (eds) (1985) *Unemployment and Health: Resources, information, action, discussion* (Glasgow: Greater Glasgow Health Board Health Education Department) (2nd revised edition, 1987).

Black, T. (1981) 'No jobs link with ill health', *Health and Social Service Journal*, Nov. 12: 1380.

Bloor, D. (1973) 'Wittgenstein and Mannheim on the sociology of mathematics', *Studies in the History and Philosophy of Science*, 4: 173–91.

Bloor, D. (1976) *Knowledge and Social Imagery* (London: Routledge and Kegan Paul).

Blume, S. S. (1987) 'Social science in Whitehall', in M. Bulmer (ed.) 1987.

Booth, T. A. (1982) 'Economics and the poverty of social planning', *Public Administration*, 60: 197–214.

Booth, Tim (1988) *Developing Policy Research* (Aldershot: Avebury).

Booth, A. E. and A. W. Coats (1978) 'The market for economists in Britain 1945–1975 – a preliminary survey', *Economic Journal*, 88: 436–54.

Boreham, J. (1984a) 'Official statistics in troubled times: the changing environment for producers and users', *Statistical News*, 64: 1–3.

Boreham, J. (1984b) 'The Central Statistical Office', *Statistical News*; 65: 1–5

Boreham, J. (1985) 'Integrity in the Government Statistical Service', *Statistical News*, 68: 19–20.

Brenner, M. H. (1979) 'Mortality and the national economy: a review and the experience of England and Wales 1936–1976' *The Lancet*; ii: 568–73.

Brenner, M. H. (1983) 'Mortality and economic instability: detailed analysis for Britain and comparative analyses for selected industrialized countries', *International Journal of Health Services*, 13: 563–620.

Brenner, M. H. (1987a) 'Economic instability, unemployment rates, behavioral risks, and mortality rates in Scotland, 1952–1983', *International Journal of Health Services*, 17: 475–87.

Brenner, M. H. (1987b) 'Relation of economic change to Swedish health and social well-being, 1950–1980', *Social Science and Medicine*, 25: 183–95.

Brenner, M. H. and A. Mooney (1982) 'Economic change and sex-specific cardiovascular mortality in Britain', *Social Science and Medicine*, 16: 431–42.

Brenner, M. H. and A. Mooney (1983) 'Unemployment and health in the context of economic change', *Social Science and Medicine*, 17: 1125–38.

Bulmer, M. (1978) 'Social science research and policy making in Britain' in M. Bulmer (ed.) *Social Policy Research* (London: Macmillan).

Bulmer, M. (1982) *The Uses of Social Research: Social investigation in public policy-making* (London: Allen and Unwin).

Bulmer, M. (1983) 'Using social science research in policy-making: why are the obstacles so formidable?', *Public Administration Bulletin*, 42: 37–48.

Bulmer, M. (1986) *Social Science and Social Policy* (London: Allen and Unwin).

Bulmer, M. (ed.) (1987 *Social Science Research and Government – Comparative Essays on Britain and the United States* (Cambridge: Cambridge University Press).

Butler, J. R. and M. S. B. Vaile (1984) *Health and Health Services* (London: Routledge and Kegan Paul).

Cairncross, A. (1968) 'The role of an economic adviser', *Public Administration*, 46: 1–11.

Cairncross, A. (1970) 'Economists in government', *Lloyds Bank Review*, 95: 1–18.

Callon, M. (1981) 'Boites noires et operations de traduction', *Economie et Humanisme*, 262: 53–9.

Callon, M. (1986) 'Domestication of the scallops and the fishermen of St Brieuc Bayd: some elements of the sociology of translation', in J. Law (ed.) *Power, Action and Belief* (London: Routledge and Kegan Paul).

Callon, M. and J. Law (1982) 'On interests and their transformation: enrolment and counter-enrolment', *Social Studies of Science*, 12, 615–25.

Callon, M., Law, J., and A. Rip (1986) *Mapping the Dynamics of Science and Technology* (London: Macmillan).

Cauliffe, S. V. (1976) 'Presidential address to the Royal Statistical Society', *Journal of the Royal Statistical Society* series A, 139: 1–11.

Chandler G. (1984) 'The role of statistics in keeping politicians honest', *The Professional Statistician*, 3: 10.

Caplan, N. (1976) 'Social research and national policy: who gets used, by whom, for what purpose and with what effects?', *International Social Science Journal*, 28: 187–94.

Carpenter, L. M. (1987) 'Some observations on the healthy worker effect', *British Journal of Industrial Medicine*, 44: 289–91.

Cherns, A. (1979) *Using the Social Sciences* (London: Routledge and Kegan Paul).

Charlton, J. R. H., Bauer, R., Thakore, A., Silver, R., and M. Aristidou (1987) 'Unemployment and mortality: a small area analysis', *Journal of Epidemiology and Community Health*, 41: 107–13.

Clarke, M. G. and H. M. Drucker (1978) *Our Changing Scotland* (Edinburgh: Edinburgh University Press).

Cochrane, A. L. (1972) *Effectiveness and Efficiency: Random Reflections on Health Services* (London: Nuffield Provincial Hospitals Trust).

Cohen, D. K. and Garet, M. (1975) 'Reforming educational policy with applied social research', *Harvard Educational Review*, 45: 17–43.

Cole, T. J., Donnet, M. L., J. P. Stansfield (1983) 'Unemployment, birth weight, and growth in the first year', *Archives of Disease in Childhood*, 58: 717–22.

Collins, H. M. (1981) 'The place of the "core set" in modern science: social contingency with methodological propriety in science', *History of Science*, 19: 6–19.

Collins, H. M. (1983) 'The sociology of scientific knowledge: studies of contemporary science', *Annual Review of Sociology*, 9: 265–85.

Collins, H. M. (1985) *Changing Order* (London: Sage).

Collins, H. R., and T. J. Pinch (1979) 'Construction of the paranormal – nothing unscientific is happening', *Sociological Review Monograph No. 27*, 237–70.

Committee of the Privy Council on Medical Research (1949) *Report of the MRC for the Years 1945–1948* (Cmnd. 7846) (London: HMSO).

Cook, D. G. (1985) 'A critical view of the unemployment and health debate', *The Statistician*, 34: 73–82.

Cook, D. G. Cummins, R. O., Bartley, M. J., and A. G. Shaper (1982) 'Health of unemployed middle aged men in Great Britain', *The Lancet*, i: 1290–94.

Cook, D. G., and A. G. Shaper (1985) 'Unemployment and health' in J. M. Harrington (ed.) *Recent Advances in Occupational Health, Volume II* (Edinburgh: Churchill Livingstone).

Cooke, K. (1988) 'The costs of unemployment', in R. Walker, and G. Parker (eds) *Money Matters* (London: Sage).

Coutouzis M. and B. Latour (1986) 'Le village solaire de Frangocastello: towards an ethnography of contemporary technology', *L'Annee Sociologique*, 36: 114–66.

Crawford, M., Morris, J. N. and J. A. Heady (1961) 'Hardness of water supplies and mortality from cardiovascular disease in the county boroughs of England and Wales', *The Lancet*, i: 860–2.

Crick, B. (1982) *In Defence of Politics*, 2nd edition (Harmondsworth: Penguin)

Culyer, A. J. (1976) *Need and the National Health Service* (London: Martin Robertson).

Daniel, W. W. (1983) 'How the unemployed fare after they find new jobs', *Policy Studies*, 3: 246–60.

Deacon, A. (1976) 'In search of the scrounger', *Occasional Papers in Social Administration*, No. 6 (London: G. Bell and Sons).

Deacon, A. (1978) 'The scrounging controversy: public attitudes toward the unemployed in contemporary Britain', *Social and Economic Administration*, 1978: 12.

Deacon, A., and R. A. Sinfield (1977) 'The unemployed, policy and public debate: the significance of the scrounging controversy', (paper to SSRC Workshop on Social Security, 18 March).

Department of Health and Social Security (DHSS) (1972) *Management Arrangements in the Reorganised NHS (The 'Grey Book')* (London: HMSO).

DHSS (1980) *Inequalities in Health – Report of a Working Group* (London: DHSS).

DHSS (1983) *Handbook of Research and Development* (London: HMSO).

DHSS (1984) *Handbook of Research and Development* (London: HMSO).DHSS (1985) *Handbook of Research and Development* (London: HMSO).

Ditch, J. (1986) 'The undeserving poor: unemployed people, then and now', in M. Loney (ed.) *The State or the Market* (London: Sage).

Doll R. (1967) 'Epidemiology', *Medical Research Council Annual Report* April 1966–March 1976 (London: MHSO).

Downs, A. (1973) 'Up and down with ecology', in J. Bains (ed.) *Environmental Decay* (Boston: Little, Brown).

Doyle, W. Hare, W. R., and M. A. Crawford (1982) 'Comparisons of fatty acid intakes in contrasting socio-economic groups during pregnancy', *Proceedings of the Nutrition Society*; 42: 69A–70A

Draper, P. and T. Smart (1974) 'Social science and health policy in the United Kingdom: some contributions of the social sciences to the bureaucratisation of the National Health Service', *International Journal of Health Services*, 4: 453–70.

Draper, P. and A. Scott-Samuel (1986) 'Whatever happened to public health?', *Health and Social Service Journal*, 26 March: 322.

Drucker H. M. and G. Brown (1980) *The Politics of Nationalism and Devolution* (London: Longman).

Durbin, J. (1987) 'Statistics and statistical science (Presidential address)' *Journal of the Royal Statistical Society* series A, 150: 177–91.

Engelman, S. (1980) 'Health economics, health economists, and the NHS', *Community Medicine*, 2: 126–34.

Eyler, J. M. (1979) *Victorian social medicine: the ideas and methods of William Farr* (Baltimore: Johns Hopkins University Press).

Fagin, L. (1981) *Unemployment and Health in Families: Case studies based on family interviews* (London: DHSS).

Fagin, L. and M. Little (1985) *The Forsaken Families* (London: Penguin).

Farrow, S. (1983) 'Monitoring the health effects of unemployment', *Journal of the Royal College of Physicians of London*, 17: 99–105.

Feldstein, M. S. (1967) *Economic Analysis for Health Service Efficiency* (Amsterdam: North-Holland Publishing Company).

Fevre R. (1986) 'Contract work in the recession' in K. Purcell, S. Wood, A. Waton, and S. Allen (eds) *The Changing Experience of Employment* (London: Macmillan).

Fevre, R. (1987) 'Subcontracting in steel', *Work, Employment and Society*, 1: 509–27.

Field, F. (1982) 'The minimum needs of children', in F. Field (ed) *Poverty and Politics* (London: Heinemann).

Flather, P. (1987) 'Pulling through – conspiracies, counterplots, and how the SSRC escaped the axe in 1982', in M. Bulmer (ed) *op. cit.*

Flinn, M. W. (ed) (1965) *The Sanitary Condition of the Labouring Population of Great Britain, by Edwin Chadwick* (Edinburgh: EUP).

Florey, C. du V and J. M. Weddell (1976) 'The epidemiologist's contribution', in K. Dunnell (ed.) *Health Services Planning* (London: King Edward's Fund).

Forbes, J. F. and A. McGregor (1984) 'Unemployment and mortality in post-war Scotland', *Journal of Health Economics*, 2: 239–57.

Forbes, J. F. and A. McGregor (1987) 'Male unemployment and cause-specific mortality in postwar Scotland', *International Journal of Health Services*, 17: 233–40.

Fox, A. J. (1979) 'The contribution of the OPCS to occupational epidemiology', *Annals of Occupational Hygiene*, 21: 393–403.

Fox, A. J. (1986) *Socio-demographic origins and consequences of unemployment: a study of changes in individuals' characteristics between 1971 and 1981* (London: Social Statistics Research Unit, City University, mimeo).

Fox, A. J. (1989) *Health Inequalities in European Countries* (Aldershot: Gower).

Fox, A. J. and P. F. Collier,(1976) 'Low Mortality rates in industrial cohort studies due to selection for work and survival in industry', *British Journal of Preventive and Social Medicine*, 9: 180–5.

Fox, A. J. and P. O. Goldblatt (1982) *Socio-Demographic Differentials in Mortality: The OPCS Longitudinal Study* (London: HMSO).

Fox, A. J. and P. O. Goldblatt (1986) 'Have inequalities in health widened?', *Social Statistics Research Unit Working Paper*, no. 4 (London: City University).

Fox, D. M. (1986) 'The National Health Service and the Second World War: the elaboration of consensus', in H. L. Smith (ed.) *War and Social Change* (Manchester: Manchester University Press).

Fry, G. K. (1986) *The Administrative 'Revolution' in Whitehall* (London: Croom Helm).

Fuchs, V. (ed.) (1972) *Essays in the Economics of Health and Medical Care* (New York: Columbia University Press for National Bureau of Economic Research).

Gandy, O. (1982) *Beyond Agenda Setting* (Norwood, N. J.: Ablex).

Gilbert, G. N. and N. Mulkay (1984) *Opening Pandora's Box: a sociological analysis of scientists' discourse* (Cambridge: Cambridge University Press).

Gill, D. G. (1976) 'The reorganisation of the NHS – some sociological aspects with special reference to the role of the community physician', in M. Stacey (ed.) 'The sociology of the National Health Service', *Sociological Review Monograph* 22, (Keele, University of Keele Press).

Gillespie, B., Eva, D. and R. Johnston (1979) 'Carcinogenic risk assessment in the United States and Great Britain: the case of aldrin/dieldrin', *Social Studies of Science*, 9: 265–301.

Goldblatt, P. O. (1990) *Mortality and Social Organisation* (London: HMSO).

Goldenberg, E. (1975) *Making the Papers* (Lexington, Mass.: D. C. Heath).

Golding, P. and S. Middleton (1982) *Images of Welfare: Press and public attitudes to poverty* (Oxford: Martin Robertson).

Goldthorpe, J. H. *Social Mobility and Class Structure in Modern Britain* (Oxford: Clarendon Press).

Gravelle, H. S. E., Hutchinson, J., and J. Stern (1981) 'Mortality and unemployment: a critique of Brenner's time-series analysis', *The Lancet*, ii: 675–9.

Gravelle, H. S. E (1985) *Does Unemployment Kill?* (York: Nuffield/York Portfolio No. 9).

Gravelle H. S. E. and M. E. Backhouse (1987) 'International cross-section analysis of the determination of mortality', *Social Science and Medicine*; 25: 427–41.

Griffin, T. (ed.) (1985) 'State figures: transcript of a filmed conversation between Sir John Boreham and Sir Claus Moser', *Statistical News*, 69: 11–16.

Haberer, J. (1972) 'Politicization in science', *Science*; 178: 713–24.

Habermas, J. (1972) *Knowledge and Human Interest* (Boston: Beacon Press)

Hakim, C. (1982) 'The social consequences of high unemployment', *Journal of Social Policy*, 4: 433–67.

Hall, P., Land, H., Parker, R., and A. Webb (1978) *Change, Choice and Conflict in Social Policy* (London: Heinemann).

Ham, C. (1985) *Health Policy in Britain* (London: Macmillan).

Hannay, D. R. (1979) *The Symptom Iceberg: A study of community health* (London: Routledge and Kegan Paul).

Harris, C. C. (1987) *Redundancy and Recession in South Wales* (Oxford: Basil Blackwell).

Harris, C. C., Lee, R. M., and L. D. Morris (1985) 'Redundancy in steel: labour market behaviour, local social relations and domestic organisation' in K. Roberts, R. Finnegan and D. Gallie (eds) *New Approaches to Economic Life* (Manchester: Manchester University Press).

Harris, C. and R. Smith (1987) 'What are health authorities doing about the health problems caused by unemployment?', *BMJ*, 294 (25 April):

1076–9.

Harris, M. (1984) 'How unemployment affects people', *New Society*, 19 January: 88–90.

Harwood, J. (1979) 'Heredity, environment and the legitimation of social policy', in B. Barnes and S. Shapin (eds) *Natural Order* (London: Sage).

Harwood, J. (1980) 'Nature, nurture and politics: a critique of the conventional wisdom', in J. V. Smith and D. Hamilton (eds) *The Meritocratic Intellect: Studies in the History of Educational Research* (Aberdeen: Aberdeen University Press).

Harwood, J. (1982) 'American academic opinion and social change: recent developments in the nature–nurture controversy', *Oxford Review of Education*, 8: 41–67.

Hauser, M. M. (ed.) (1972) *The Economics of Medical Care* (London: George Allen and Unwin).

Helco, H. and A. Wildavsky (1974) *The Private Government of Public Money* (London: Macmillan).

Heller, T. (1978) *Restructuring the Health Service* (London: Croom Helm).

Hencke, D. (1986) 'Fowler sets up health inquiry', *Guardian*, 22 January.

Henderson, A. S., and C. C. Williams (1974) 'On the prevention of parasuicide', *Australia and New Zealand Journal of Psychiatry*; 8: 237–40.

Hennock, E. P. (1976) 'Poverty and social theory in England: the experience of the 1880s', *Social History*, 1: 67–91.

Himsworth, H. (1984) 'Epidemiology, genetics and sociology', *Journal of Biosocial Science*, 16: 159–76.

Hoinville, G. and T. H. F. Smith (1982) 'The Rayner review of government statistical services', *Journal of the Royal Statistical Society*, Series A, 145: 195–207.

HMSO (1981) *Government Statistical Services* ('The Rayner White Paper') Cmnd. 8236 (London: HMSO).

Holland, W. W. (1982) 'Rethinking community medicine: a reflection', *Community Medicine*, 3: 40–43.

Hughes, E. (1971) *The Sociological Eye* (Chicago: Aldine).

Hughes, P. R. and G. Hutchinson. (1986) 'Changing characteristics of male unemployment flows 1972–1981', *Employment Gazette*, September: 365–73.

Illsley, R. (1986) 'Occupational class, selection and inequalities in health', *Quarterly Journal of Social Affairs*, 2: 151–65.

Jefferys, M. (1986) 'The transition from public health to Community Medicine: The evolution and execution of a policy for occupational transformation', *Bulletin of the Society for the Social History of Medicine*, 39: 47–63.

Johnston, P. (1986) 'Letter from Westminster: Unemployment kills, claims Labour's Michael Meacher', *BMJ*, i: 1344.

Joint Working Party on the Integration of Medical Work (1973) *Community Medicine in Scotland: The 'Gilloran Report'* (Edinburgh: HMSO).

Jones, G. (1986) *Social Hygiene in Twentieth Century Britain* (London: Croom Helm).

Jones, I. G. and D. Cameron. (1983) 'John Snow, the Broad Street Pump and modern epidemiology', *Community Medicine*, 12: 393–6.

Junankar, P. N. (1986) 'Mortality and unemployment: a preliminary analysis' (University of Essex, Department of Economics Discussion Paper No. 282).

Kallen, D. B. P., Koss, G. B., Wagenaar, H. C, Kloprogge, J. J. J., and M. Vorbeck (eds) (1982) *Social Science Research and Public Policy-Making – A Re-appraisal* (Windsor, Berks: NFER-Nelson).

Klein, R. (1982) 'Performance, evaluation and the NHS: a case study in conceptual perplexity and organisational complexity', *Public Administration*, 60: 385–407.

Knorr, K. D., Krohn, R., and R. Whitley. (eds) (1980) *The Social Process of Scientific Investigation* (Dordrecht: Reidel).

Knorr-Cetina, K. (1981) *The Manufacture of Knowledge: An essay in the constructivist and contextual nature of science* (Oxford: Pergamon).

Knorr-Cetina, K. (1982) 'Scientific communities or transepistemic arenas of research? A critique of quasi-economic models of science', *Social Studies of Science*, 12: 101–30.

Kogan, M. and M. Henkel (1983) *Government and Research* (London: Heinemann).

Lambert, R. (1963) *Sir John Simon 1816–1904 and English Social Administration* (London: Macgibbon and Kee).

The Lancet (editorial) (1984) 'Unemployment and health', ii: 1018–9.

The Lancet (1986) 'Commentary from Westminster: Government's record on health', i: 923–24.

Last, J. M. (1963) 'The illness iceberg', *The Lancet*, II: 28–31.

Latour, B. (1981) 'Le chercheur aussi est un negotiateur rusé', *Economie et Humanisme*, 262: 13–17.

Latour, B. (1984a) *Les Microbes: Guerre et Paix* (Paris: Editions Métailié, Collection Pandore).

Latour, B. (1984b) A simple model for treating technoscience evolution (Paper to International Workshop of New Developments in the Social Studies of Technology, Twente).

Latour, B. (1987) *Science in Action* (Milton Keynes: Open University Press).

Latour, B. (1988) 'The politics of explanation', in S. Woolgar (ed.) *Knowledge and Reflexivity* (London: Sage).

Latour, B. and S. Woolgar (1979) *Laboratory Life* (Beverley Hills: Sage).

Latour, B. and S. Woolgar. (1986) *Laboratory Life*, second edition (Princeton, New Jersey: Princeton University Press).

Laurence, J. (1986) 'How ministers fiddle figures', *New Society*, 28 February: 361.

Law, J. (1983) 'Enrolement et contre-enrolement: les luttes pour la publication d'un article scientifique', *Social Science Information*, 22: 237–51.

Law, J. (1986) 'On the methods of long-distance control: vessels, navigation and the Portuguese route to India' in J. Law (ed.) *Power, Action and Belief* (London: Routledge and Kegan Paul).

Ledwith, F. (1987) 'Lest we forget the common good', *Health Service Journal*, 30 April: 500–501.

Lee, R. M. (1985) 'Redundancy, labour markets and informal relations', *Sociological Review*, 33: 469–95.

Leete, R. and Fox, J. (1977) 'Registrar General's social classes: origins and uses' *Population Trends*, 8: 1–7.

Le Grand, J. (1987) 'Health and wealth' *New Society*, 16 January: 9–11.

Lewis, J. (1986a) *What Price Community Medicine?* (Brighton: Wheatsheaf).

Lewis, J. (1986b) 'The changing fortunes of community medicine', *Public Health* 100: 3–10.

Lindblom, C. (1979) 'Still muddling, not yet through', *Public Administration Review*, 39: 517–26.

Linton, M. (1987) 'When conscience is put to the vote', *Guardian*; 16 January: 5.

London School of Hygiene and Tropical Medicine (1968) *Report of the Work of the School 1967–8* (London: LSHTM).

London School of Hygiene and Tropical Medicine (1969) *Report of the Work of the School* (London: LSHTM).

Lynch, M. E. (1982) 'Technical work and critical inquiry: investigations in a scientific laboratory', *Social Studies of Science*, 12: 499–533.

MacAvinchey, I. D. (1984) 'Unemployment and mortality: some aspects of the Scottish case 1950–1978', *Scottish Journal of Political Economy*, 31: 827–33.

McCarthy, M. (1986) *Campaigning for the Poor* (London: Croom Helm).

Macdonagh, O. (1958) 'The nineteenth-century revolution in government: a reappraisal', *The Historical Journal*, 1: 52–67.

Macdonagh, O. (1961) *A Pattern of Government Growth* (London: Macgibbon and Kee).

McKee, L. and C. Bell (1986) 'His unemployment, her problem: the domestic and marital consequences of male unemployment', S. Allen, A. Waton, K. Purcell, and S. Woods (eds.) *The Experience of Unemployment* (London: Macmillan).

Mackenzie, D. (1981a) *Statistics in Britain 1865–1930: The Social Construction of Scientific Knowledge* (Edinburgh: Edinburgh University Press).

Mackenzie, D. (1981b) 'Interests, positivism, and history', *Social Studies of Science*, 11: 498–504.

McKeown, T. (1976) *The Modern Rise of Population* (London: Arnold).

McKeown, T. (1979) *The Role of Medicine* (London: Nuffield Provincial Hospitals Trust).

McKeown, T. and C. R. Lowe (1966) *An Introduction to Social Medicine* (Oxford: Blackwell).

Macleod, R. M. (1967) 'The frustration of State medicine', *Medical History*, 11: 15–40.

McMahon, L., Barrett, H. S., and M. Hill (1983) 'Power bargaining models in policy analysis, *Public Administration Bulletin*, 43: 49–68.

Manning, N. (ed.) (1985) *Social Problems and Welfare Ideology* (London: Gower).

Martin, F. M. (1977) 'Social medicine and its contribution to social policy', *The Lancet*, ii (24–31 Dec): 1336–8.

Martin, R. (1987) 'A new realism in industrial relations?', in S. Fineman (ed.) *Unemployment – Personal and Social Consequences* (London: Tavistock).

Medical Research Council (1957) *Annual Report* (London: HMSO).

Medical Research Council (1959) *Annual Report* (London: HMSO).

Medical Research Council (1970) *Annual Report* (London: HMSO).

Medical Research Council (1974) *Annual Report* (London: HMSO).

Medical Research Council (1975) *Annual Report* (London: HMSO).

Medical Research Council, Unit for Epidemiological Studies in Psychiatry (1964) *Progress Report* (Edinburgh, mimeo).

Medical Research Council, Unit for Epidemiological Studies in Psychiatry (1974) *Progress Report* (Edinburgh, mimeo).

Metcalfe, L. and S. Richards (1987) *Improving Public Management* (London: Sage).

Micklewright, J. (1986) 'Unemployment and incentives to work: policy and evidence in the 1980s', in P. E. Hart (ed.) *Unemployment and Labour Market Policies* (Aldershot: Gower).

Moon, J. and J. J. Richardson (1984) 'The unemployment industry', *Policy and Politics*; 12: 391–411.

Morrell, D. C. and C. J. Wale (1976) 'Symptoms perceived and recorded by patients', *Journal of the Royal College of General Practitioners*, 26: 398–403.

Morris, J. N. (1964) *Uses of Epidemiology* (London: Churchill Livingstone).

Morris, J. N. and R. Titmuss (1944) 'Health and social change: recent history of rheumatic heart disease', *The Medical Officer*: 69–71, 77–9, 85–7.

Morris, J. N. (1971) 'Tomorrow's community physician', in A. Gatherer and M. D. Warren (eds) *Management and the Health Services* (London: Pergamon).

Moser, C. A. (1973) 'Staffing in the government statistical service', *Journal of the Royal Statistical Society*, series A, 136: 75–88.

Moser, C. A. (1980) 'Statistics and public policy', *Journal of the Royal Statistical Society*, series A, 143: 1–32.

Moser, K. A., Fox, A. J., and D. R. Jones (1984) 'Unemployment and mortality in the OPCS Longitudinal Study', *The Lancet*, ii: 1324–9.

Moser, K. A., Goldblatt, P. O., Fox, A. J., and D. R. Jones (1987a) 'Unemployment and mortality, 1981–83: follow-up of the 1981 Census sample', *BMJ*, 294: 86–90.

Moser, K. A., Goldblatt, P. O., Fox A. J., and D. R. Jones (1987b) 'Unemployment and mortality', (letter) *BMJ*, 294: 509.

Moser, K. A., Goldblatt, P. O., Fox, A. J., and D. R. Jones (1987c) 'Unemployment and mortality', (letter) *BMJ*, 294: 153.

Moylan, S., Millar, J., and R. Davies (1984) *For Richer, For Poorer: DHSS Cohort Study of Unemployed Men DHSS Research Report No. 11* (London: HMSO).

Mulkay, M., Pinch, T., and M. Ashmore (1987a) 'Colonizing the mind: dilemmas in the application of social science', *Social Studies of Science*, 17: 231–56.

Mulkay, M., Ashmore, M., and T. Pinch (1987b) 'Measuring the quality of life, a sociological invention concerning the application of economics to health care', *Sociology*, 21: 541–64.

Narendranathan, W., Nickell, S., and D. Metcalfe (1985) 'An investigation into the incidence and dynamic structure of sickness and unemployment in Britain, 1965–1975', *Journal of the Royal Statistical Society*, series A, 148: 254–67.

Nelkin, D. (1975) 'The political impact of technical expertise', *Social Studies of Science*, 5: 35–54.

Novak, S. J. (1972) 'Professionalism and bureaucracy: English doctors and the Victorian public health administration', *Journal of Social History*, 6: 440–62.

Nowotny, H., and H. Hirsch (1980) 'The consequences of dissent: sociological reflections on the controversy over low dose effects', *Research Policy*, 9: 278–94.

Office of Population Censuses and Surveys (1973) 'Cohort studies – new developments', *Report on Medical and Population Subjects*, No. 25 (London: HMSO).

Office of Population Censuses and Surveys (1978) *Occupational Mortality: the Registrar-General's Decennial Supplement for England and Wales 1970–1972* (London: HMSO).

Office of Population Censuses and Surveys (1986) *Occupational Mortality: Decennial Supplement 1979–80, 1982–83* (London: HMSO).

Opie, R. (1968) 'The making of economic policy', in H. Thomas (ed.) *Crisis in the Civil Service* (London: Anthony Blond).

Orchard, T. (1985) 'Government statistics in the 1980s: a half term report', *Statistical News*, 68: 9–12.

Parker, R. (1983) 'Research and the politics of comparison' in J. Gandy, A. Robertson, and S. Sinclair (eds) *Improving Social Intervention* (Edinburgh: Edinburgh University Press).

Parston, G. (1980) *Planners, Politics and Health Services* (London: Croom Helm).

Perlman, M. (1974) *The Economics of Health and Medical Care* (London: Macmillan).

Petersen, J. C. and G. E. Markle (1981) 'Expansion of conflict in cancer controversies', *Research in Social Movements, Conflict and Change*, 4: 151–69.

Pfautz, H. (1967) *Charles Booth and the City: Physical Pattern and Social Structure* (University of Chicago Press)

Pinch, T. and W. E. Bijker (1984) 'The social construction of facts and artefacts: or how the sociology of science and the sociology of technology might benefit each other', *Social Studies of Science*, 14: 399–441.

Platt, S. (1982) 'Unemployment and suicide', *Unemployment Unit Bulletin*, 6: 4–8.

Platt, S. (1983) 'Unemployment and parasuicide ("attempted suicide") in Edinburgh 1968–1982', *Unemployment Unit Bulletin*, 10: 4–5.

Platt, S. (1984) Unpublished Ph D, Edinburgh University. Results summarised in 'A subculture of parasuicide?', *Human Relations*, 38:257–97.

Platt, S. (1986a) 'Recent trends in parasuicide ("attempted suicide") and unemployment among men in Edinburgh', in S. Allen, A. Waton, K. Purcell, and S. Wood (eds) *The Experience of Unemployment* (London: Macmillan).

Platt, S. (1986b) 'Parasuicide and unemployment', (Annotation) *British Journal of Psychiaty*, 149: 401–405.

Platt, S. and N. Kreitman (1984) 'Trends in parasuicide among men in Edinburgh 1968–1982', *BMJ*, 289: 1029–32.

Platt, S. and N. Kreitman (1985) 'Parasuicide and unemployment among men in Edinburgh 1968–1982', *Psychological Medicine*, 15: 113–23.

Pollert, A. (1987) 'The "flexible firm": a model in search of reality', *Warwick Papers in Industrial Relations* no. 19 (Warwick: University of Warwick, Industrial Relations Research Unit).

Popay, J. (1977) 'Fiddlers on the Hoof – moral panics and social security scroungers.', dissertation, MA in Social Service Planning (Essex: University of Essex).

Porter, A. M. D. (1979) 'Measurement: Health economics – models, achievements and limitations', in K. M. Boyd (ed.) *The Ethics of Resource Allocation* (Edinburgh: Edinburgh University Press).

Porter, D. (1990) 'How soon is now?, Public Health and the *British Medical Journal*', *BMJ* 301, 738–40.

Posner, M. (1982) 'Review of the SSRC', *SSRC Newsletter*, 46: 1–5.

Prentice, T. (1987) 'Jobless men facing higher risk of death, says survey', *The Times*, 9 January, p. 4.

Prince, M. J. (1983) *Policy Advice and Organisational Survival: Policy planning and research units in British government* (Aldershot: Gower).

Ramsden, S. and C. Smee (1981) 'The health of unemployed men: DHSS Cohort Study', *Employment Gazette*, 89: 397–401.

Rayner, B. (1977) 'The DHSS research arrangements', *SSRC Newsletter*, 35: 4–11.

Rayner Report (1980) *Sir Derek Rayner's report to the Prime Minister* (London: HMSO).

Reader, W. J. (1966) *Professional Men* (London: Wiedenfeld and Nicholson).

Rein, M. (1980) 'Interplay between social science and social policy', *International Social Science Journal*, 32: 361–8.

Rein, M. (1983) *From Policy to Practice* (New York: M. E. Sharpe).

Reubens, B. (1970) *The Hard-to-Employ: European Programs* (Columbia University Press)

Richardson, J. J. and A. G. Jordan (1979) *Governing Under Pressure* (Oxford: Martin Robertson).

Rothschild, L. (1982) *An Enquiry into the Social Science Research Council* Cmnd, 8554 (London: HMSO).

Royal Statistical Society (1968) 'British official statistics: a discussion held before the RSS', *Journal of the Royal Statistical Society*, series A, 131: 1–8.

Russell E. M. (1984) 'Choice and change in health care in Britain', *Social Science and Medicine*, 18: 27–40.

St George D. (1985) 'Managers attempt to hijack community medicine', *BMJ*, 291: 1589–90.

Salter, H. C. (1972) 'Public expenditure and the health and welfare services', in Hauser (ed.) 1972.

Scambler, A., Scambler, G., and D. Craig (1981) 'Kinship and friendship networks and women's demand for primary care', *Journal of the Royal College of Physicians*, 31: 746-50.

Scott, A. (1988) 'Imputing beliefs: a controversy in the sociology of knowledge', *Sociological Review*, 36: 41–57.

Scott-Samuel, A. (1985) 'Does Unemployment Kill?' (letter) *British Medi-*

cal Journal, 290: 1905.

Joint Working Party on the Integration of Medical Work, Scottish Home and Health Department (1973) *Community Medicine in Scotland: The 'Gilloran Report'* (Edinburgh: HMSO).

Seaton, J. (1986) 'The media and the politics of interpreting unemployment' in S. Allen, A. Waton, K. Purcell, and S. Wood (eds) *The Experience of Unemployment* (London: Macmillan).

Shapin, S. (1982) 'History of science and its sociological reconstruction', *History of Science*, 20: 157.

Shapin, S. (1988) 'Following scientists around, Review of *Science in Action*', *Social Studies of Science*, 18: 532–50.

Sharpe, L. J. (1978) 'Government as clients for social science research', in M. Bulmer (ed.) *Social Policy Research* (London: Macmillan).

Shils, E. (1961) 'The calling of sociology', in T. Parsons, E. Shils, K. D. Naegele, and J. R. Pitts (eds) *Theories of Society* (New York: Free Press).

Sinfield, R. A. (1981) *What Unemployment Means* (Oxford: Martin Robertson).

Sinfield, R. A. (1987) 'Unemployment experience and policy responses in overseas countries', paper to conference on Income Support and Labour Market Change, Department of Social Security, Canberra, September 1987.

Smith, A. R. (1984) 'The Department of Health and Social Security', *Statistical News*, 67: 5–13.

Smith, B. S. (1987) 'Unemployment and mortality' (letter) *BMJ*, i: 509.

Smith, C. (1987) 'Networks of influence: the social sciences in Britain since the war', in M. Bulmer (ed.) *op. cit.*

Smith, R. (1985) 'Bitterness, shame, emptiness, waste: an introduction to unemployment and health', *BMJ*, ii: 1024–7.

Smith, R. (1986a) 'The need for a Public Health Alliance', *BMJ*, 293 (9 Aug): 346–7.

Smith, R. (1986b) 'Long live health promotion', *BMJ*, 293 (6 Dec): 1457–8.

Smith, R. (1987a) 'More evidence on unemployment and health', *BMJ*, 294 (25 April: 1047–8.

Smith, R. (1987b) *Unemployment and Health: A Disaster and a Challenge* (Oxford: Oxford University Press).

Smith, M. (1979) 'Community Medicine: a speciality in its death throes?', *World Medicine*, 10 February:

Social Services Select Committee (1981) *House of Commons Papers, Session 1980–1981*, HC 324–II, 12 May 1981.

Spector, M. and J. I. Kitsuse (1977) *Constructing Social Problems* (Menlo Park, California: Cummings).

Stern, J. (1979) 'Who bears the burden of unemployment?', in W. Beckermann (ed.) *Slow Growth in Britain* (Oxford: Clarendon Press).

Stern, J. (1982) 'Does unemployment really kill?', *New Society*, 10 June: 421–2.

Stern, J. (1983a) 'Social mobility and the interpretation of social class mortality differentials', *Journal of Social Policy*, 12: 27–49.

Stern, J. (1983b), 'The relationship between unemployment, morbidity and mortality, in Britain', *Population Studies*, 37: 61–74.

Strong, P. M. (1979) 'Sociological imperialism and the profession of medicine – a critical examination of the thesis of medical imperialism', *Social Science and Medicine*, 13A: 199–215.

Times Health Supplement, Editorial (1982) 'Out of work, out of sorts', *Times Health Supplement* 29 October: 412–3.

Tizard, B. (1990) 'Research and policy: is there a link', *The Psychologist*, 10: 435–40.

Travis, A. (1985) 'Senior Whitehall men sidelined', *Guardian*, 12 November.

Unit for the Study of Health Policy (1979) *Rethinking Community Medicine* (London: USHP).

Wagstaff, A. (1986a) 'The demand for health, a simplified Grossman model', *Bulletin of Economic Research*, 38: 93–5.

Wagstaff, A. (1986b) 'The demand for health – new empirical evidence', *Journal of Health Economics*, 5: 195–233.

Wagstaff, A. (1986c) 'Unemployment and health: some pitfalls for the unwary', *Health Trends*; 79–81.

Walker, A., Noble, I., and J. Westergaard (1985) 'From secure employment to labour market insecurity: the impact of redundancy on older workers', in B. Roberts, R. Finnegan, and D. Gallie (eds) *New Approaches to Economic Life* (Manchester: Manchester University Press).

Walker, R. (1987) 'Perhaps, Minister: the messy world of "in-house" social research', in M. Bulmer (ed.) 1987.

Watkins, D. E. (1984) *The English Revolution in Social Medicine 1889–1911* (PhD thesis, London: University of London).

Watkins, D. E. (1986) 'What was social medicine? A historiography of the concept (or, George Rosen revisited)', *Bulletin of the Society for the Social History of Medicine*, 38: 47–51.

Webster, C. (1982) 'Healthy or hungry "Thirties?"', *History Workshop Journal*, 13: 110–29.

Webster, C. (1986) 'The origins of social medicine in Britain', *Bulletin of the Society for the Social History of Medicine*, 38: 52–5.

Weinerman, E. R. (1951) *Social Medicine in Western Europe* (Berkeley, California: University of California Press).

Weiss, C. H. (1979) 'The many meanings of research utilisation', *Public Administration Review*, 39: 426–32.

Weiss, C. H. (1982) 'Policy research in the context of diffuse decision-making', in D. B. P. Kallen, G. B. Kosse, H. C. Wagenaar, J. J. J. Kloprogge, and M. Vorbeck (eds) *Social Science Research and Public Policy Making – A Reappraisal* (Windsor, Berks: NFER-Nelson).

Westcott, G. M., Svensson, P-G, and H. Zollner (eds) (1985) *Health Policy Implications of Unemployment* (Copenhagen: WHO Regional Office for Europe).

Westcott, G. (1987) 'The effects of unemployment on health in Scunthorpe and related health risk factors', *Public Health*, 101: 399–416.

White, M. (1983) *Long Term Unemployment and Labour Markets* (London, Policy Studies Institute).

Whitehead, F. (1984) 'The Office of Population Censuses and Surveys', *Statistical News*, 66:

Whitely, P. and S. Winyard. (1983) 'Influencing social policy: the effectiveness of the poverty lobby in Britain', *Journal of Social Policy*, 12: 1–26.

Whitely, P. and S. Winyard (1984) 'The origins of the "new poverty lobby"', *Political Studies*, 32: 32–54.

Whiteside, N. (1987) 'Counting the cost: sickness and disability among working people in an era of industrial recession, 1920–1939', *Economic History Review*, 40: 228–46.

Whiteside, N. (1988) 'Unemployment and health: an historical perspective', *Journal of Social Policy*, 17: 177–94.

Whitley, R. (1972) 'Black boxism and the sociology of science: a discussion of major developments', in P. Halmos (ed.) *The Sociology of Science* (London; Routledge and Kegan Paul).

Whitley, R. (1982) 'The establishment and structure of the sciences as reputational organisations', in N. Elias, H. Martins, and R. Whitley (eds) *Scientific Establishments and Hierarchies* (Dordrecht: Reidel)

Wilkinson, R. G. (1986) *Class and Health: Research and Longitudinal Data* (London: Tavistock).

Wilkinson, R. G. (1990) 'Income distribution and mortality: a "natural" experiment', *Sociology of Health and Illness*, 12: 391–412.

Wohl, A. S. (1983) *Endangered Lives* (London: Dent).

Woolgar, S. (1981) 'Interests and explanations in the social study of science', *Social Studies of Science*, 11: 365–94.

Woolgar, S. and D. Pawluch (1985a) 'Ontological gerrymandering: the anatomy of social problems explanations', *Social Problems*, 32: 214–27.

Woolgar, S. and D. Pawluch (1985b) 'How shall we move beyond constructivism?', *Social Problems*, 33: 159.

INDEX